Better Homes and Gardens®
Your Baby GROWS UP

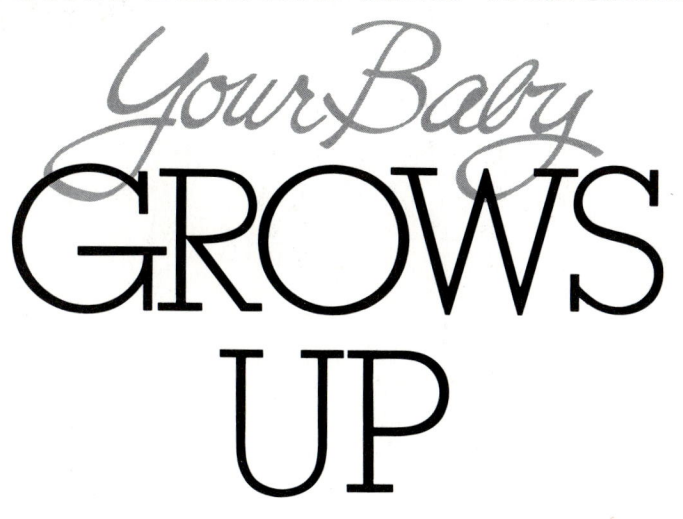

18 Months–6 Years

By Edwin Kiester, Jr., and Sally Valente Kiester
and the Editors of Better Homes & Gardens® Books

Photography by
Kathryn Abbe and Frances McLaughlin-Gill

Excerpted from the Better Homes and Gardens® NEW BABY BOOK

BETTER HOMES AND GARDENS® BOOKS
Editor: Gerald M. Knox
Art Director: Ernest Shelton
Managing Editor: David A. Kirchner
Editorial Project Managers: James D. Blume, Marsha Jahns, Rosanne Weber Mattson, Mary Helen Schiltz
Associate Art Directors: Linda Ford Vermie, Neoma Alt West, Randall Yontz
Assistant Art Directors: Lynda Haupert, Harijs Priekulis, Tom Wegner
Senior Graphic Designer: Darla Whipple-Frain
Graphic Designers: Mike Burns, Brian Wignall
Art Production: Director, John Berg; Associate, Joe Heuer; Office Manager, Emma Rediger

President, Book Group: Fred Stines
Vice President, General Manager: Jeramy Lanigan
Vice President, Retail Marketing: Jamie Martin
Vice President, Administrative Services: Rick Rundall

BETTER HOMES AND GARDENS® MAGAZINE
President, Magazine Group: James A. Autry
Vice President, Editorial Director: Doris Eby
Executive Director, Editorial Services: Duane L. Gregg

MEREDITH CORPORATE OFFICERS
Chairman of the Board: E.T. Meredith III
President: Robert A. Burnett
Executive Vice President: Jack D. Rehm

YOUR BABY GROWS UP
Editorial Project Manager: Mary Helen Schiltz
Graphic Designer: Lynda Haupert
Electronic Text Processor: Paula Forest

ACKNOWLEDGMENTS
Jack E. Obedzinski, M.D., Assistant Clinical Professor of Pediatrics, Child Study Unit, University of California, San Francisco; Center for Families and Children, Corte Madera, California.
D. Stewart Rowe, M.D., Associate Clinical Professor of Pediatrics, University of California, San Francisco.

© Copyright 1987 by Meredith Corporation, Des Moines, Iowa. All Rights Reserved. Printed in the United States of America.
First Edition. First Printing.
ISBN: 0-696-01723-7

CONTENTS

EIGHTEEN MONTHS TO
    TWO YEARS 5

TWO TO THREE YEARS 15

THREE TO FIVE YEARS 25

FIVE TO SIX YEARS 39

MEDICAL RECORDS CHART 45

BABY RECORDS 46

INDEX 48

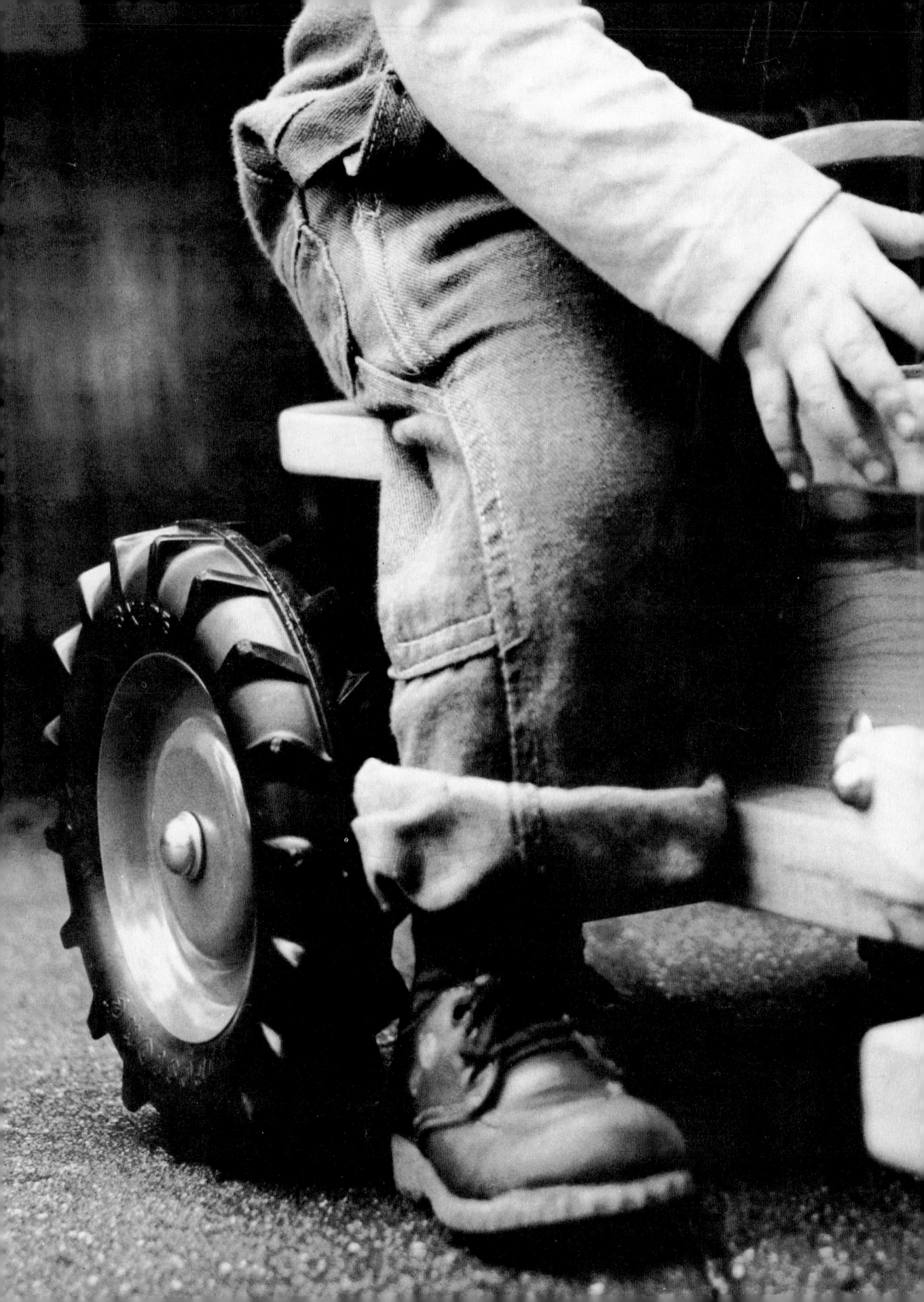

EIGHTEEN MONTHS TO TWO YEARS

HOW THE BABY GROWS

The growth rate slows considerably during the last half of the baby's second year. The average normal two-year-old weighs 28 pounds and is 34½ inches tall. The range for normal babies is 23½ to 32½ pounds and 32 to 36½ inches.

Here are some things normal babies learn to do between 18 and 24 months:
• use words in combination to make simple statements or questions;
• identify one or more parts of the body;
• follow simple directions—most of the time—if only a single step is involved;
• put on some items of clothing—but try more than succeed;
• wash and dry their hands, with parental supervision;
• identify pictures of animals by name;
• build a tower of eight blocks;
• pedal a tricycle; propel a kiddie car with feet;
• kick a ball forward or throw it overhand, neither with accuracy.

THE ART OF CONVERSATION

A two-year-old's communication is no longer limited to a few semi-intelligible words, noises, grunts, and gestures. Vocabulary increases, pronunciation improves, and the patterns of adult speech begin. The number of words—and ideas—the baby comprehends grows dramatically.

The baby may begin to speak in sentences (although many normal babies do not combine words for another year). They're not complex, adult statements and questions: just two words put together to express basic wants and thoughts. At first, sentences will consist of just a noun and a verb, without much respect for the niceties of grammar: "Fred eat," "Mommy stay," "Go bye-bye." There will be simple questions, too: "Where Doggie?" "Who that?" But in a surprisingly short time, your son or daughter will be stringing together three or even four words into an understandable combination.

Meanwhile, as many parents are amazed (and pleased) to learn, the baby "understands everything you say!" "Passive" vocabulary grows so greatly that you can now communicate ideas that a few weeks or months ago were totally over the child's head. "Let's go in the car," you'll say, and Rachel or Ted will dash for the door—obvious proof the message has been understood. You can give simple commands or directions, confident they will be carried out: "It's time for lunch," and the baby will head for the high chair or eating table. You may even find yourself in a parent-to-child dialogue complete with statements and responses:

"Who toy?" "That's Jennifer's toy."
"Where J'fer?"
"Want cookie." "No cookies until lunch."
"Want cookie!"

Of course, developmental rates are erratic. Children vary in how quickly they master communication skills. Some shy, quiet children don't add words so quickly or roll them off the tongue so glibly as more outgoing, energetic personalities (although temperaments aren't always a key to verbal ability). Even the most verbally precocious may develop vocabulary in a spurt, slow down for a few weeks or months, then take another great leap forward. Girls are thought to be more fluent than boys the same age. Children in some families are more verbal than children in other families, but even children in the same family may not master speech at the same rate.

You'll find the baby has quite a storehouse of knowledge. An average 21-month-old can correctly identify one or more parts of the body. Ask, "Where is Adam's nose?" "Where is Adam's hand?" and a stubby finger may accurately point to the named part, perhaps accompanied by the emphatic declaration, "Nose!" "Hand!" or even "Adam hand!" A child nearing his or her second birthday may be able to point to the baby, horse, or dog in a book. Most children this age can tell you their names. Family members now are all identified by name, usually with a highly personal pronunciation.

Now that the child's speech has improved, you may find that behavior and disposition improve, too. There may be fewer tantrums and temperamental outbursts when your son or daughter is able to tell you what he or she wants. You may even be able to reason with the child when things don't seem to go the right way. And the baby will now have a say in the family's affairs, not simply be a passive listener.

You can help your child develop language at this stage just by talking to him or her. In fact, you'll probably find yourself doing so almost unconsciously, just to watch the responses. "Time for lunch," you'll say, and plop him or her into the high chair. Your comments and conversations help the child to learn new words, as well as the purposes of oral communication. When you give commands or directions to a child, try to see they are carried out to strengthen the concept that words have meaning.

TIME FOR OUTDOOR PLAY

Your offspring is now ready for more play outdoors. Depending on where you live and the size of your purse, you may wish to establish his or her own area in the yard or on the porch. If a parent is home during the day, the best location is directly outside a window where you can keep an eye on the child and he or she can be aware of your presence.

The play area need not be large. A space 15 by 20 feet allows plenty of room to roam. The play area should be completely enclosed, with a gate latch that resists little fingers or is beyond their reach, so you can feel free to leave the child alone.

For play equipment, a small sandbox complete with pails, shovels, spoons, and other digging implements is basic. If the baby can climb, a small slide is inexpensive fun. Swings will come a little later, although you may wish to install an entire "outdoor gym" at once. You can sometimes find these at garage sales or secondhand stores, although you should check them carefully for safety features. For almost no money, you can equip the area with boxes, cubes, discarded tires, and even old tree stumps for the child to climb on, crawl over, or tunnel through. Falls will be frequent, so a grassy surface or sand is best.

Your son or daughter also is ready for more advanced toys. A few two-year-olds can pedal a tricycle or miniature auto; younger children can manipulate a kiddie car or other vehicle propelled with the feet. Indoors, a rocking horse can provide hours of fun, and building blocks become an important part of the toy chest.

If you live in an apartment or haven't room for your own play area, take the child to a park or playground often: Space to run freely is important at this age. Neighborhood parks usually have a fenced toddlers' area with special equipment. Occasional supervised visits to a wading pool, lake, or seashore also are fun. But don't let the child play on the sidewalk or in an unconfined area outside the house.

TIME FOR PLAYMATES

More and more, your child will enjoy playing with children the same age. Children under two still don't really play together, but just watching each other is half the fun. Put a pair of two-year-olds side-by-side in a sandbox, and each will dig his or her own hole, fill his or her own bucket, and push his or her own truck, but there will be a good deal of pausing, observing, mimicking, and imitating. Also, toys will be grabbed, snatched, and passed back and forth. Pushing and shoving are part of the routine.

Not much time will be wasted by two-year-olds on the niceties of language, but you'll be surprised at how effectively the two youngsters manage to communicate with each other.

Some children plunge right into social situations and enjoy them; others take time to warm up. Your child may not feel comfortable with more than one playmate at a time; playground noise may be frightening. A shy, quiet child may hang back and cling to parents or be much more content to play alone within sight of the others, gradually working into the group. Other children may use the bull-in-a-china-shop approach. They may hit, poke, bite, or grab toys without giving them back. Such encounters between two-year-olds often are accompanied by a great deal of crying and complaining.

Within the limits of safety, you should try to keep hands off and let the children work things out for themselves; the tussles aren't really arguments. If one child pushes another, the second is likely to push back: the message is conveyed in a primitive way that pushing is unpopular and should be stopped. If you move in to end things too quickly and retaliation isn't allowed to take place, the aggressor doesn't have a chance to learn the consequences of aggressive behavior. In fact, your child may actually be encouraged to hit because you are inadvertently protecting him or her.

If one child continues to act aggressively and the other doesn't strike back but runs away or cries and whimpers, you may be obliged to step in. If your child is the aggressor, speak firmly and sharply in disapproving tones. If the other child is the fighter, first you may have to negotiate with the child's parents. It may be necessary to separate the children.

Relationships between children often are more difficult for the parents than for the youngsters themselves. If another child repeatedly bullies your child, you may have to bring up the matter tactfully with the other parent. Parental standards differ, and it is sometimes hard for a child who has had clear, precise training to deal with a child who has not. In fact, you'll often find the other parent is giving the child a double message, vicariously enjoying the youthful aggression, while ostensibly disapproving. If so, you may have to soft-pedal the relationship with the other parent, rather than continually subject your child to a relationship that he or she is not able to handle.

LEARNING TO DRESS

The first step in dressing takes place when the child learns to name the items of clothing and the parts of the body they cover. The process of putting on clothes is usually too much for an 18-month-old, but you can begin the educational process now. Start by naming each garment as you put it on, and then send the child to get it from the drawer or closet.

Next, enlist the child's cooperation. Teach him or her how to poke feet into trousers or hold hands in the air so a sweater can be pulled over the head. You can make a game of it: "Where is Susan?" as the shirt goes over the head; "There she is!" Finally, as your child approaches two years of age, he or she can begin to put on certain items of clothing under your supervision.

At first, it's really play; the child is just imitating adult behavior. Not much is accomplished beyond pulling on socks or shoes or worming into a jacket. You'll have to show how things go on or they'll wind up backward, upside down, sideways or twisted, with shoes on the wrong feet. You'll also do the fastening. Buttons and zippers are still too much for little fingers; the small muscles haven't matured enough to allow that kind of dexterity. Even so, the child will be delighted with the dressing accomplishment.

Don't expect too much of the child at this point. The objective is really to let him or her play at the idea of dressing and learn about clothes at the same time. Patiently let the child fumble with buttons or tug at shorts; don't step in too speedily to help. Eventually, of course, you'll have to do it, after allowing a brief, tolerable period for the child's education. But be sure to praise the child's efforts.

Patient supervision applies to more lessons than dressing. You'll have to show restraint in many things as your child grows older, so he or she can learn independently.

A SENSE OF ORDER

Because the child likes to imitate grown-ups, it's now easy for you to begin helping him or her acquire a sense of order. As you work about the house, get the baby to help you with the less complicated projects at hand. At first, of course, it's only play for the baby and may be a little extra for you, but the lesson will carry over into taking care of the child's own possessions.

When you teach in this way, simplify the child's needs. Install low hooks and hangers in closets and bedrooms so clothing can be reached easily. Assign specific places for jackets, shoes, and rain gear. At first, the child will be able to do little more than retrieve the garment from the hook when you ask for it. But once the notion is clear that clothes go in a specific place, it will be easier to teach him or her to hang them or put them away later.

The child's play area should have its own storage spaces—drawers, boxes, and shelves—to hold toys. Make a nightly ritual of helping the child put the toys away for the next day's play. Of course, he or she can't do it independently at this age, but you're building a solid foundation for later behavior.

Teach the child to wash and dry hands, too. Again, training comes fairly easily because a child under two likes to imitate grown-ups. Buy a low stool or box so he or she can reach the faucet, and give him or her a personal towel, hung at an appropriately low height. Children usually prefer cool water, and you shouldn't expect a high standard of cleanliness at this point. Right now, the basic lesson is just to show how the procedure works. Teach the child to wash and dry hands before each meal—but you should expect to remind him or her for the next two or three years.

At this age, children don't really play together. But they do react to their companions. Watch closely and you'll see each observing the actions of the other and then trying them on for size.

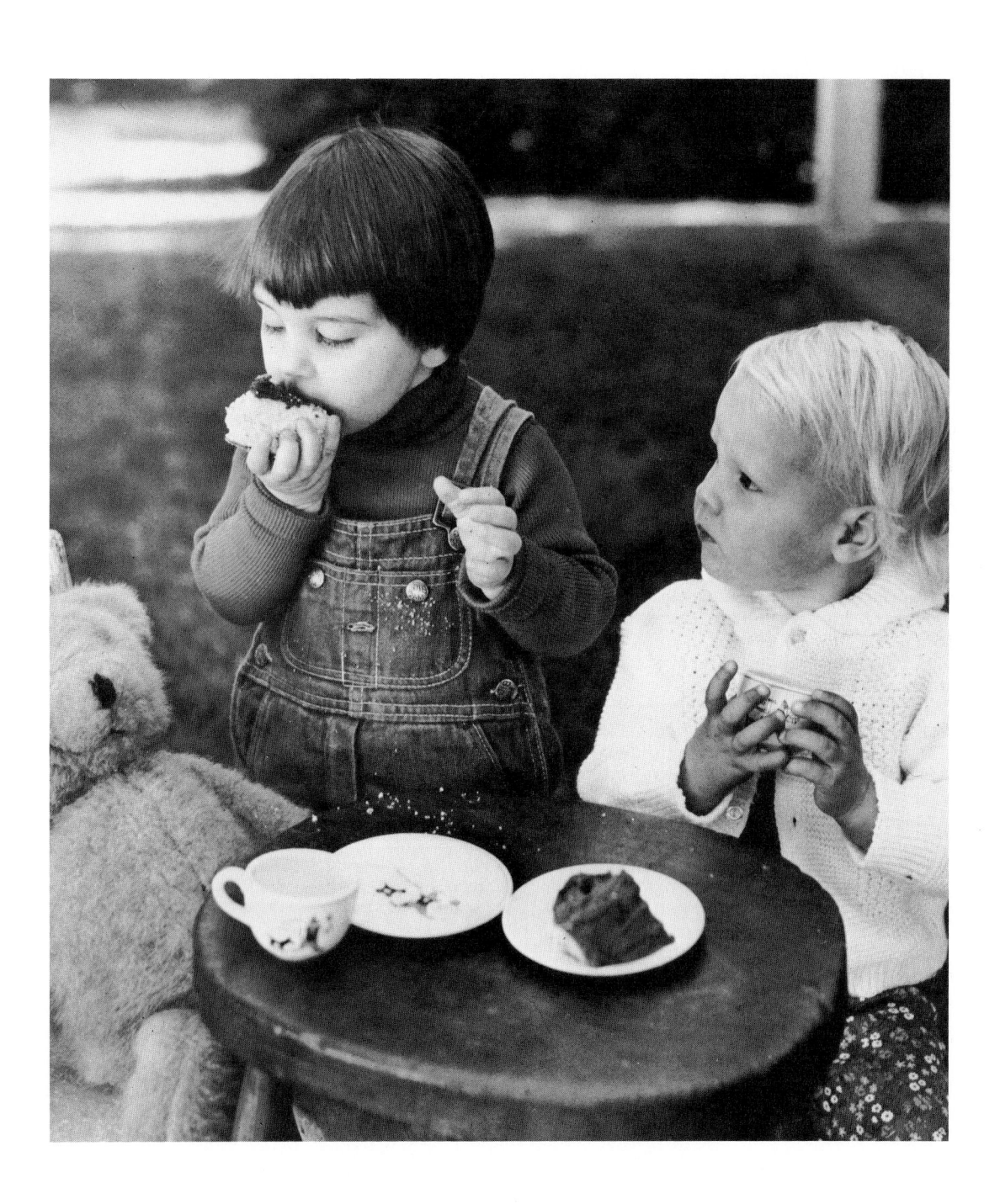

TAKING CARE OF THE TEETH

With 16 to 20 teeth, the two-year-old is more than ready for a toothbrush and a program of dental hygiene. Again, natural mimicry helps to establish good habits. Buy a small brush for the child and his or her own toothpaste and cup. At first you must hold the brush to demonstrate how it's done. The child will quickly get the idea and want to take over. Allow him or her to do so under your supervision. Of course, a child this age can't brush adequately, and you'll have to finish up after he or she has fun with the brush.

It's true the so-called baby teeth will be lost and replaced by permanent teeth, but that doesn't mean their care should be neglected. The American Dental Association (ADA) recommends the child's first dental checkup be conducted as soon as 16 baby teeth have appeared, or by the age of three, when the child can cooperate with the dentist. The ADA points out that cavities in the baby teeth or the loss of them can cause the child's permanent teeth to be pushed out of alignment. Orthodontia or other corrective measures may be necessary later. The ADA suggests a regular checkup each year after the child's first one and that dental work be done, if necessary.

Prevention, of course, is the most important ingredient of good dental care. Cavities now are recognized to be of bacterial origin; bacteria in the mouth combine with sugars, remaining on or between the teeth to produce an acid that destroys tooth enamel and eats into the heart of the tooth. Although some families seem to be more cavity-prone than others, limiting the amount of sugar can reduce cavities in many children. For better teeth, restrict chewing gum, cookies, ice cream, and sweet desserts. When sweets are eaten, the teeth should be brushed immediately, if possible, to remove the sugars that cause decay. When brushing is not convenient, the mouth should at least be rinsed with water. At the very least, the child who has eaten sweets should have his or her teeth brushed before going to bed and should not be allowed food in the crib.

The practice of letting the baby go to bed with a bottle can be potentially harmful to cavity-prone youngsters, especially if the baby keeps the bottle in the mouth throughout the night or sucks on it periodically. Sugars in formula, milk, or juice, not normally damaging, thus bathe the teeth constantly and promote tooth decay. No harm seems to result when the baby drinks for a short period and the bottle is discarded or removed by parents.

If the water supply in your community is not fluoridated, your doctor or dentist may prescribe fluoride supplements for the child's teeth. These are recommended by both the ADA and the American Academy of Pediatrics.

Although not so effective as fluoridated water in preventing decay, these treatments include using chewable fluoride tablets, allowing the dentist to paint the teeth with fluoride, and brushing with fluoridated toothpaste.

EATING PROBLEMS

The picky appetite continues. There are two related reasons: the child eats less because the rate of growth has slowed and less food is needed; and the body slims as the supply of baby fat is used up, so that contours begin to resemble those of an adult. Mother and father observe and conclude the child isn't eating enough. Result: they try to push more food on the child, the child resists, and each meal increasingly resembles a power struggle.

The most sensible and straightforward rule for feeding at this stage is simple: observe how much the child ordinarily eats; serve approximately that quantity or a bit more; try to balance out the nutrients over a period of time (but not necessarily at one meal or even in one day); offer three main meals a day, with a cracker or cookie in midmorning and midafternoon.

At mealtimes, let the child decide how much is enough. When he or she seems to have lost interest, try offering one more bite. If it's not accepted, take the food away and let the child leave the high chair or table.

Given a choice, most children prefer sweets to other foods, so you'll have to work hard to keep him or her from concentrating on sweet desserts while neglecting other foods. There's probably no way to avoid sugar completely, but do your best to limit the child's intake of refined sugar to protect the teeth. Perhaps you can restrict it to plain cookies or simple desserts. An occasional treat, of course, is fine. Good ice cream is a nourishing food readily eaten by young children.

READY FOR TOILET TRAINING

There's no set schedule for toilet training. Most parents expect to begin when their youngster is about 18 months of age, but the child, not the calendar, tells you when the time is right. Logically, there is little point in trying until the child recognizes that he or she is having a bowel movement and can communicate that fact to you. There's wide variation as to when recognition and communication occur; even when they do, many children simply aren't interested in bowel training—they have better things to do! Studies show that four out of five normal children are daytime-trained by 2½ years, but some haven't mastered the technique by the age of four.

Of course, some parents boast of a child who was bowel-trained at a year of age, or even earlier. What this usually means, however, is that the *parent* was trained. Having observed that the child had a bowel movement at a regular time each day, the alert mother or father placed the baby on the potty at the appropriate hour and "caught" the movement. The mystified child usually had no idea what he or she was doing.

When you feel your child is nearly ready for training, buy a small potty chair for the child to use. A freestanding chair with removable potty is usually better than a seat that fits the standard toilet, because it's closer to the ground and the child won't be afraid of falling or of the flushing noise. Also, you can move the potty chair to where you are, instead of isolating the child in the bathroom.

Every family has its own words for the need to urinate or defecate. It's important for a child to use these words to tell you (or if you ask) when it's time to use the toilet.

Long before the child does, you'll probably notice the bowel movements follow a pattern. That's not true of all children: some are wildly irregular and may have a movement only every few days, making training more difficult. But most children have a daily movement; a common time is just after breakfast, apparently because the reflexive movements within the intestines resume their normal daytime pace. A few children have two or more movements a day.

Once you've discovered the appropriate time, place the baby on the potty chair for a short period as that hour approaches. Don't make the stay too long, and don't, by any means, strap the child in place. If the child produces a movement, be sure to praise the effort, so the message is clear the purpose of sitting has been fulfilled. If nothing happens, allow the child to leave the chair when he or she wants to.

Some children will sit for a time without results, then have a movement immediately after standing up. The association is clear; the timing is off. In cleaning up, try to be as matter-of-fact as you can. Remembering the child's growing vocabulary, explain that movements are to be made in the potty and that being clean is nicer than being soiled. Repeat the message when it's time to change soiled diapers. Suggest the child tell you if he or she wishes to use the potty.

READY FOR URINE TRAINING

Bowel training may be accomplished within a few days or weeks, but some months will pass before the child is reliable and motivated to use the toilet. Urine training takes even longer and may be marked by long efforts without success. Urine training usually follows bowel training by up to six months. At first, sitting down is usually the appropriate posture for urination—for boys as well as girls.

The first clue that it's time for urine training comes when you notice the child's diapers remain dry for longer periods during the day, perhaps for two hours or more at a time. This usually happens some time after 18 months of age. That's because the bladder has grown and has a larger storage capacity. It also indicates the beginning of control over the bladder.

Teaching a child under two how to wash and dry hands is fairly easy. Though your son or daughter won't become proficient at it right away, the basic procedure—to be followed before and after meals—is the important lesson.

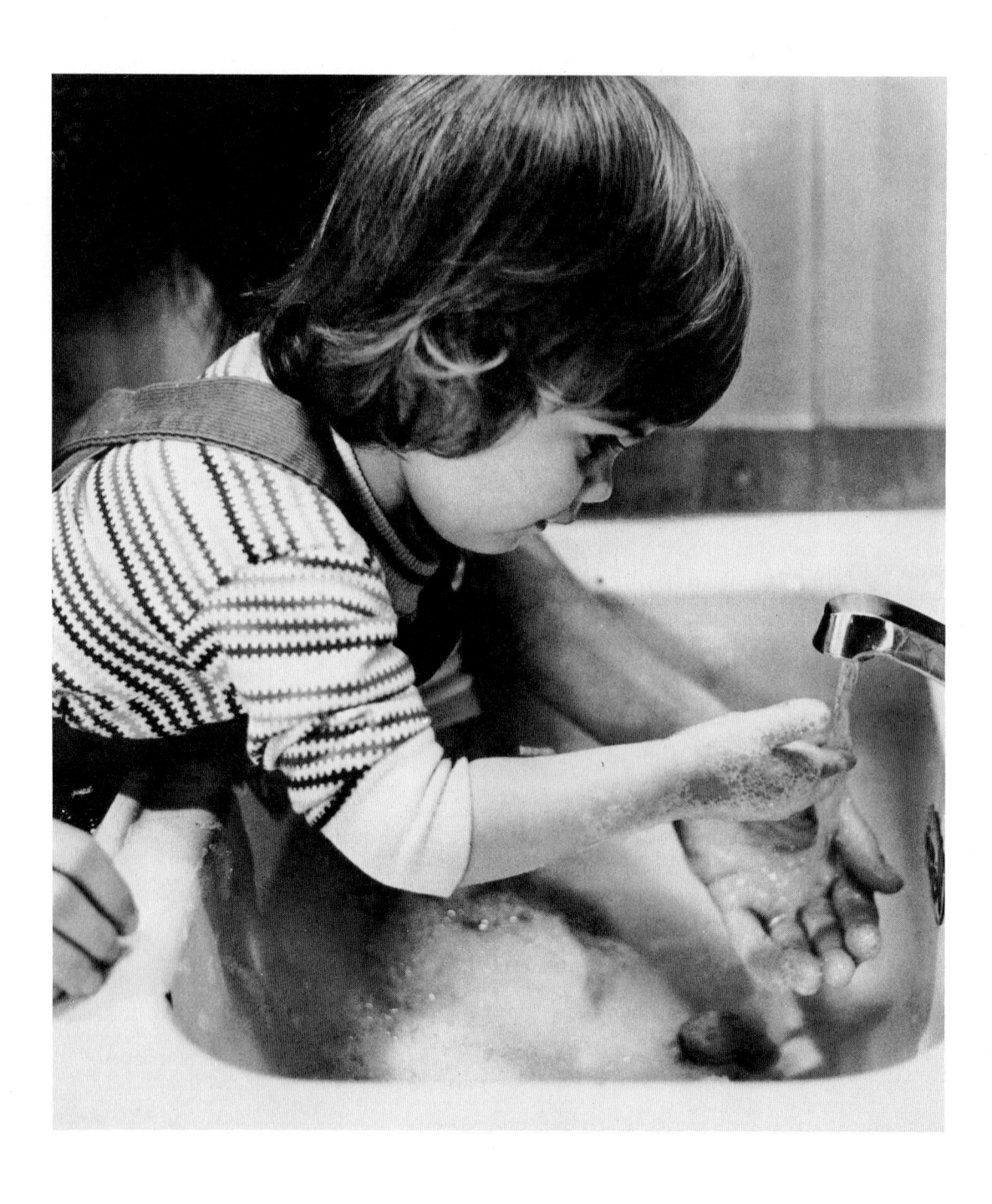

Another clue comes from the child. He or she may come to you after urinating and complain of wet diapers. The child may even hold the crotch or tug at the diaper, either before or after urinating. Again, the child's timing is off, but there's a clear association between wet diapers and the act of urinating. It also indicates the child is beginning to feel uncomfortable when wet, a fact you can take advantage of when urging him or her to urinate in the potty.

Once you're aware of these indications, begin placing the child on the potty at approximately two-hour intervals. Before and after naps, at mealtimes, and at bedtime are appropriate moments. You'll have to set the schedule for a while. The child isn't likely to be aware that he or she is ready to urinate until the last minute. As with bowel movements, the child will often urinate after leaving the potty.

Complete control of the bladder takes time to develop; once a child's bladder is full, he or she may not be able to wait even another minute to empty it. Also, boys in particular may have a more difficult time retaining urine. Some boys can't hold back urine for more than two hours until age three.

Remember, you'll also have to teach the child the proper words to tell you when he or she needs to urinate.

Training pants instead of diapers are helpful, once the baby can stay dry for two or more hours. They're not only simpler to put on and take off, but they have the psychological advantage of being "grown-up." Some doctors believe that babies feel free to urinate in diapers, whereas they exercise greater control while wearing training pants.

KEEPING THINGS CASUAL

Although many people regard it otherwise, toilet training needn't be a big deal. Like other aspects of child-rearing, training isn't a competition, and years from now, it'll make little difference that you had to launder diapers for six more months than the parents next door. Patience on your part is as important to the baby's toilet training as bladder control. You may experience a long stretch without success, even though the child clearly understands the task; nothing is so annoying to parents as when they ask, "Do you have to wee-wee?" and the child solemnly denies it, while the puddle grows around his or her feet. Exasperating as the drawn-out procedure may be, scolding, shaming, or demanding immediate and perfect results doesn't help to keep diapers dry. In any case, the baby has the ultimate weapon. Nothing you can do or say will cause him or her to urinate or defecate (or withhold it) if he or she doesn't want to.

ACCIDENTS AND BREAKDOWNS

Even after the child is reasonably well trained, accidents will happen. Stress or excitement may cause the baby to urinate; some babies can't urinate on an unfamiliar potty and will wet their pants instead. Accidental urination is more common in cold weather than in warm weather. In any case, accidents should be treated routinely—but not ignored. Mention to the child that he or she would be more comfortable with clean and dry clothing.

With some children, toilet training seems to go fine for a while, then collapses. The child will return to earlier habits; you may even feel compelled to use diapers again. Often, there's an obvious reason: when a new child enters the household, for instance, an older child may revert to babyish practices. Sometimes, though, no reason can be discerned.

When that happens, treat the setback as calmly as possible. You may even drop toilet training for a time, return the child to diapers, and wait. Usually, the child will independently disclose a new readiness for further training. If the child simply balks at using the toilet at the times or places you suggest, let him or her pick the times. Sometimes, the child simply hasn't achieved full muscular control. He or she may be unable to relax while sitting on the toilet but may be able to relax while standing. But, if possible, avoid making toilet training an issue. It's a battle no parent can win.

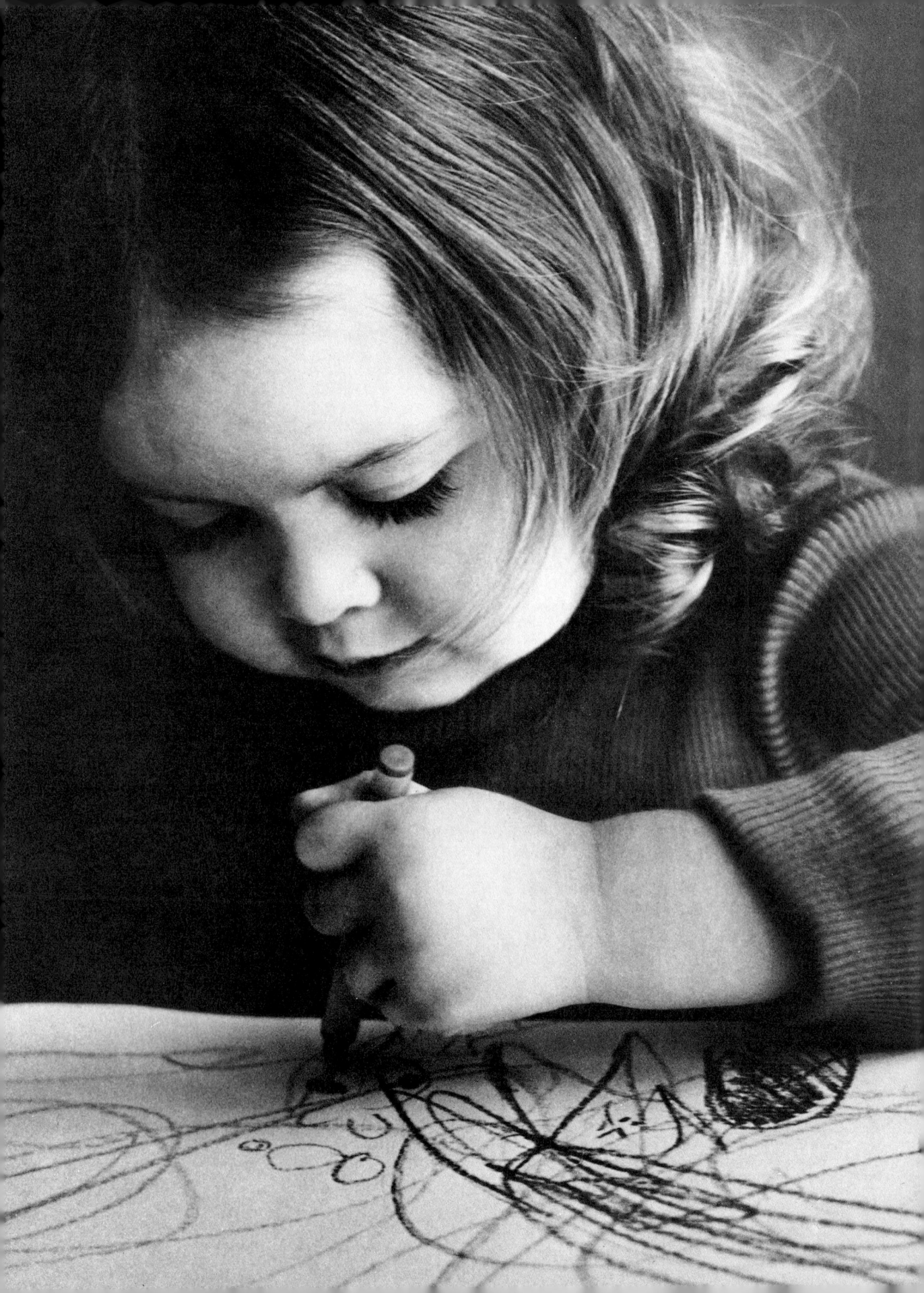

TWO TO THREE YEARS

HOW THE CHILD GROWS

Between the second and third birthdays, the average normal child gains four pounds and grows 3½ inches. Average weight for a three-year-old boy is 32½ pounds; average height, 38 inches; for girls, 31 pounds and 37 inches. The range for normal children is 25½ to 38 pounds and 35 to 40½ inches.

Here are some things half of the normal children learn to do between the ages of two and three:
- dress with supervision and button some buttons;
- play interactive games, such as hide-and seek;
- tell their own first and last names;
- use plurals, pronouns, and prepositions in speech;
- copy a circle with a crayon;
- understand such words as "cold," "tired," and "hungry";
- know where things belong and help to put them there;
- follow simple directions;
- feed themselves almost completely;
- be toilet-trained during the day and remain dry all night some of the time;
- recognize and identify some colors.

INCREASING SELF-RELIANCE

Day by day through the third year of life, children grow more self-reliant. Each new adventure makes them more conscious of their own individuality, their own control over their minds and bodies. Independence increases. They learn to do many things for themselves—after a fashion, at least—and, indeed, insist on it. The statement "Me do it" is familiar to any parent.

Feeding will be strictly a "do-it-myself" project, as it should be. The child's style of eating will still lack finesse, and at the completion of a meal, the table may resemble San Francisco after the earthquake. Watery soups and runny puddings will still defeat the novice eater; sandwiches will continue to be dissected before they're digested. But he or she is much better coordinated than a year ago. And with a full complement of teeth, the child can now eat firmer foods that previously were withheld, such as breadsticks.

Skill in dressing will improve steadily. As any parent can tell you, at first a two-year-old's attempts to put on clothes are little more than play, humorous imitations of what grown-ups do. Most of the actual routine of dressing a child falls to the parents. But as the months pass, your child will become more adept at wriggling into a playsuit or pulling on socks. A three-year-old may even laboriously manage a few buttons, even if the correct button doesn't match the proper buttonhole. Ironically, as mastery improves, the child loses interest in what is no longer a hill to climb—but a tedious chore.

You'll continue to establish the child's routine of eating, sleeping, and playing, but the child will want some voice in it. He or she will want to play when he or she wants to play and may stubbornly state the case with emphatic words and gestures. For your own convenience and the child's welfare, you may have to be firm.

Increasingly, your role becomes more that of model than nurse. You demonstrate, the child imitates, you correct and help. Some of the imitations are just for fun at first. But you may be astonished at the amount of time and concentration your child will devote to mastering some simple task, like pedaling a kiddie car, as he or she continues to seek new worlds.

THE LITTLE MONARCH

The two-year-old is a creature of moods, too. One of them is a kind of haughty, regal manner that is insistingly self-indulgent. With all the imperiousness of Napoleon or Catherine the Great, the two-year-old monarch will boss everybody—parents, siblings, domestic animals—and insist on having his or her own way. Nothing short of a palace revolt will overturn the royal dictum, "Gimme cookie!"

Two is also the traditional age of disobedience—although it may merely be the parents' label for the child's tendency to do as he or she pleases. It's not so much defiance; the child resents restrictions, resents limits, and doesn't want to be told what to do. "No" will be another mainstay of the vocabulary, although you'll usually hear it as "NO!" You may find yourself enforcing a number of rules with "friendly muscle" instead of "sweet reasonableness." It won't be enough to tell the child to stop doing something; you may have to physically call a halt.

Actually, you'll find a two-year-old's behavior shot full of contradictions. One day your son or daughter will be balky, contrary, cantankerous; anything you suggest will be rejected, even if it is something that delighted him or her only yesterday. Just wait: tomorrow will bring sunshine, cooperation, and agreeableness. Ann or Andrew will be a pleasure to be with. These behavioral zigzags can be exasperating to parents, who often wail, "He was so nice yesterday and so terrible today!" Consistency is simply not in the cards yet. It'll be at least a year until he or she is predictable—and closer to four before he or she obeys consistently.

All this is just another phase of growing up. The child is now learning the art of the possible—discovering the limits of behavior, what is permissible and what isn't. Still self-centered, he or she hasn't learned to distinguish between what he or she wishes would happen and what can *actually* happen. The two-year-old operates in the here and now and can't always fit present attitudes into a pattern of behavior, as an adult usually can. And many a two-year-old's attitudes really don't mean much; they're just tests. Even using the word "no" is just another way of learning what happens after saying it.

To a two-year-old, the whole world is a private kingdom where all wishes automatically come true. Parents, siblings, and small kittens will be wrapped up by the child's desire to have it "my way."

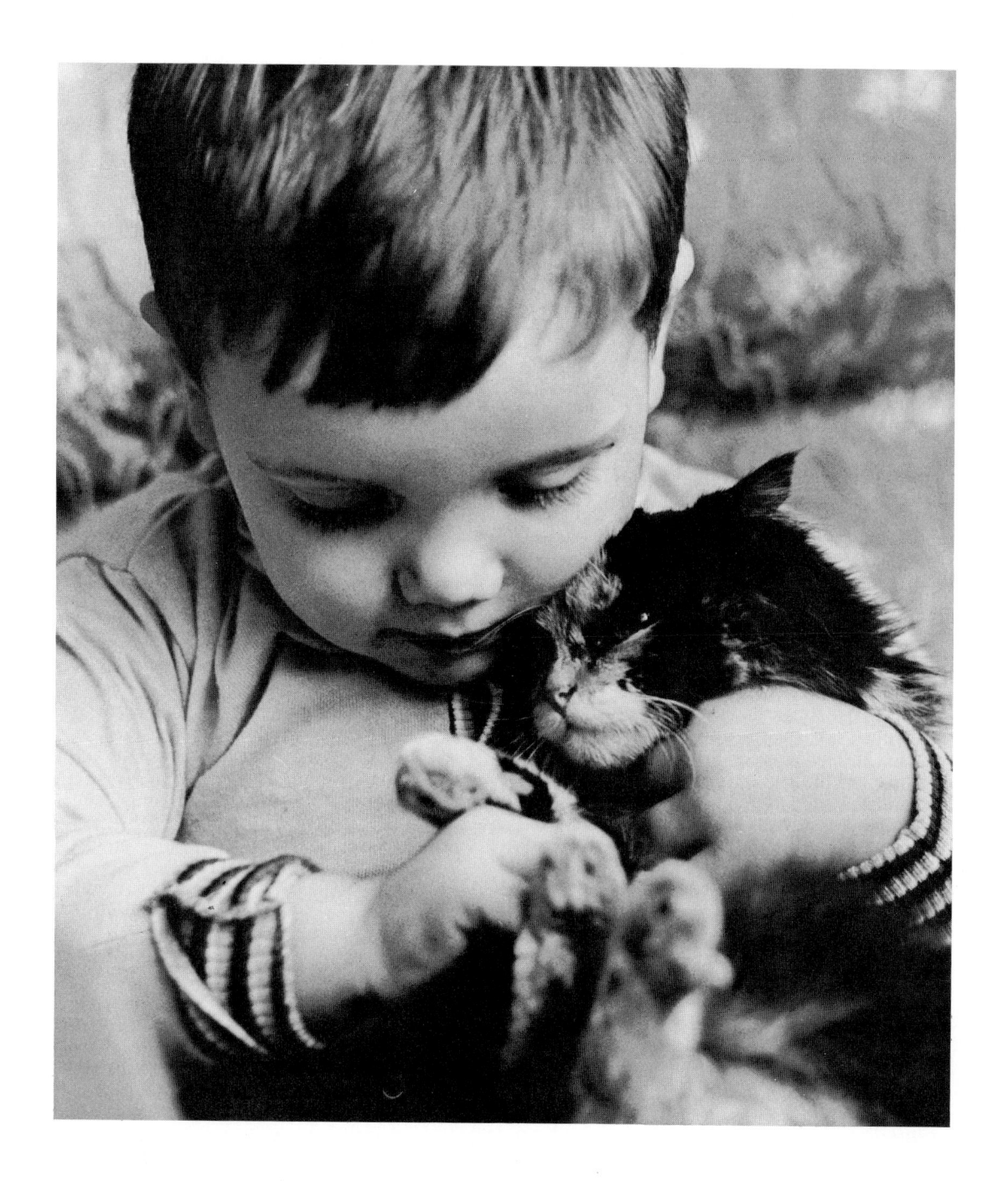

A FAVORITE PARENT

Part of a two-year-old's inconsistency may be attachment to one parent or the other. Some children cling to mother or father and openly dismiss the other. Boys usually attach themselves to fathers and girls to mothers; later, the preference may be for the parent of the opposite sex.

This, too, is just a phase and won't last. The best policy—for both parents—is to ignore this phase and ride it out.

That may be easier said than done: The rejected parent feels hurt; the favorite, defensive and guilty. Sometimes the rejected parent also tries to make up to the child and win back him or her. If so, the child may learn to play one parent against the other. Parents should stand together, unified in their approach to children; they shouldn't be sensitive about presumed shows of favoritism.

THOSE MADDENING RITUALS

With growing powers of observation and memory, a two-year-old knows and remembers where everything in the house belongs and how every act of daily routine is performed. Amazingly, he or she will even remember exactly where you're supposed to turn the car on the way to grandmother's house or which aisle you usually visit first in the supermarket. And, often to your dismay, you'll have to do everything in precisely the same manner and keep everything just as it was yesterday, the day before, and the day before that.

Lunch must always be served on the same plate. The teddy bear must always be propped in the southwest corner of the crib—moving it to the northeast will bring squalls of protest. The bedtime ritual must follow exactly the same sequence—story, drink, toilet, drink, toilet, "Night-night." Change the order, omit one step, even substitute "So long" for "Night-night," and you'll hear about it. The objections will be loud and tiringly sustained.

At age two, the world is an avalanche of novel experiences and situations slightly altered from the day before. Naturally, a young learner wants some things to count on—some things to remain reliably cemented in time while he or she moves on to new, exciting matters. From your point of view, maddening though these rituals may be, they should be accepted without complaint unless they become too long, too complicated, or too intrusive on family life.

NIGHTMARES AND NIGHT FEARS

Nightmares often begin when the child is between two and three years old. But Bobby or Barbara doesn't know they're nightmares. He or she wakes, shouting in fright, to tell you that there are monsters in the room. So far as he or she is concerned, there *are* monsters lurking over behind the dresser. To a child unable to divorce fantasy from reality, even in daylight, the monsters are real.

If nightmares and night-waking are frequent, occurring every night or two, they may indicate that something else is troubling the child—the arrival of a new baby, a move to a new house, a shift in day-care arrangements. But if they occur only occasionally, then simple reassurance is enough to deal with them. Don't reason with the frightened child, explaining there are no monsters; don't turn on the light to show him or her, because he or she knows better. On the other hand, don't support the fantasy by chasing the monsters out.

Instead, distract the child as quickly as possible. Hold and soothe him or her with reassuring words until the tears stop. Then point out the familiar surroundings to ease the fears: "There's your own pillow right here"; "There's your teddy bear. Let's put him right here beside you"; "I will be in the next room and I can hear you."

Don't fuss too much about the incident (attention to it only reinforces the impression), don't remain with the child so long that he or she awakens fully, and don't transfer the child to your bed; the switch may be the beginning of a pattern of nightly awakenings. If the child recalls the incident the following night and expresses fears about staying in the room, you may wish to install a night-light for reassurance.

PLAYMATES AND PLAY GROUPS

The company of peers is no longer just a casual part of childish life. If your son or daughter is not already mingling with contemporaries in a day-care center, you should arrange for regular companionship and stimulation of others the same age.

Two-year-olds still play individually, rather than together, but cooperation and interaction—still sprinkled with shoving, pushing, and grabbing—steadily increase as the third birthday approaches. It's fun for parents to watch this stage, for three-year-olds' play is heavily laced with imagination and fantasy.

Your child may be fortunate enough to have playmates in the neighborhood, even a few steps away. If another two- or three-year-old is next door, the two may be together nearly all day, scampering back and forth between the houses and play areas without adult escort.

In an urban area or a neighborhood with few children, you'll have to schedule playtime. It needn't be an elaborate or formal arrangement, just an exchange of visits with a friend whose child is about the same age.

Or you may wish to set up a scheduled play group, whose members arrive to play at established times and places.

City parents often shepherd their children to a playground at a set time each day, knowing that other children the same age will probably be on hand. Often, the occasion is a social get-together for the parents, as well as a playtime for the children. In suburbs, a kaffeeklatsch may serve the same purpose. You and your friends can set a regular time to assemble with the children and rotate the meeting place.

Another informal arrangement resembles a baby-sitting cooperative. Two or three children gather at John's home one day, Martha's another, and Linda's a third. The designated parent supervises the children that day.

As the children grow a little older, some play groups begin to resemble preschool sessions. One parent is assigned to supervise the children at each gathering and to provide a program. This is usually something simple: a trip to the playground, paints and paper for fingerpainting, clay for modeling.

Charitable, governmental, and commercial organizations also sponsor play groups. These usually are more formal than those at child-care facilities and may be supervised by a certified specialist in early-childhood education. Some are operated in conjunction with an adult-education course in child development. Play groups also are operated (for a fee) in many cities and suburbs.

There aren't many rules to remember when establishing your own play group. Try to choose children of approximately the same age and temperament, children who are likely to stimulate each other and blend well together. The choice of adults is important, too. You want other parents whom you like and in whom you feel confidence. You'll also want to inquire discreetly about the other homes—if there's enough space for two or three boisterous three-year-olds, and whether normal safety precautions are observed.

Two hours a day, two days a week are a good beginning schedule for a play group. Children this age have a short attention span, so there should be plenty of activity to divert them. They need a good balance between physical play and crafts requiring the use of small muscles. The supervising parent may not be called upon to watch the children each minute but will have to look in regularly, referee disputes, and help the youngsters change directions. Three highly energetic three-year-olds are about as many as one parent can handle at a time; two parents can handle six or eight children.

Play groups work well when all children are about the same age, but it's also valuable for your child to have a mix of playmates. Playing occasionally with older children and occasionally with younger ones allows an opportunity both to follow and to lead. Don't segregate the sexes. Three-year-old boys and girls play equally well with each other.

IMAGINARY PLAYMATES

Often, a three-year-old's most devoted and beloved friend is invisible to everyone else. Boys and girls at three years of age often invent an imaginary playmate—human or animal—who in

Stories take children into the world of words and ideas. Keep them simple, with plenty of action and pictures. Put lots of expression and excitement into your stories.

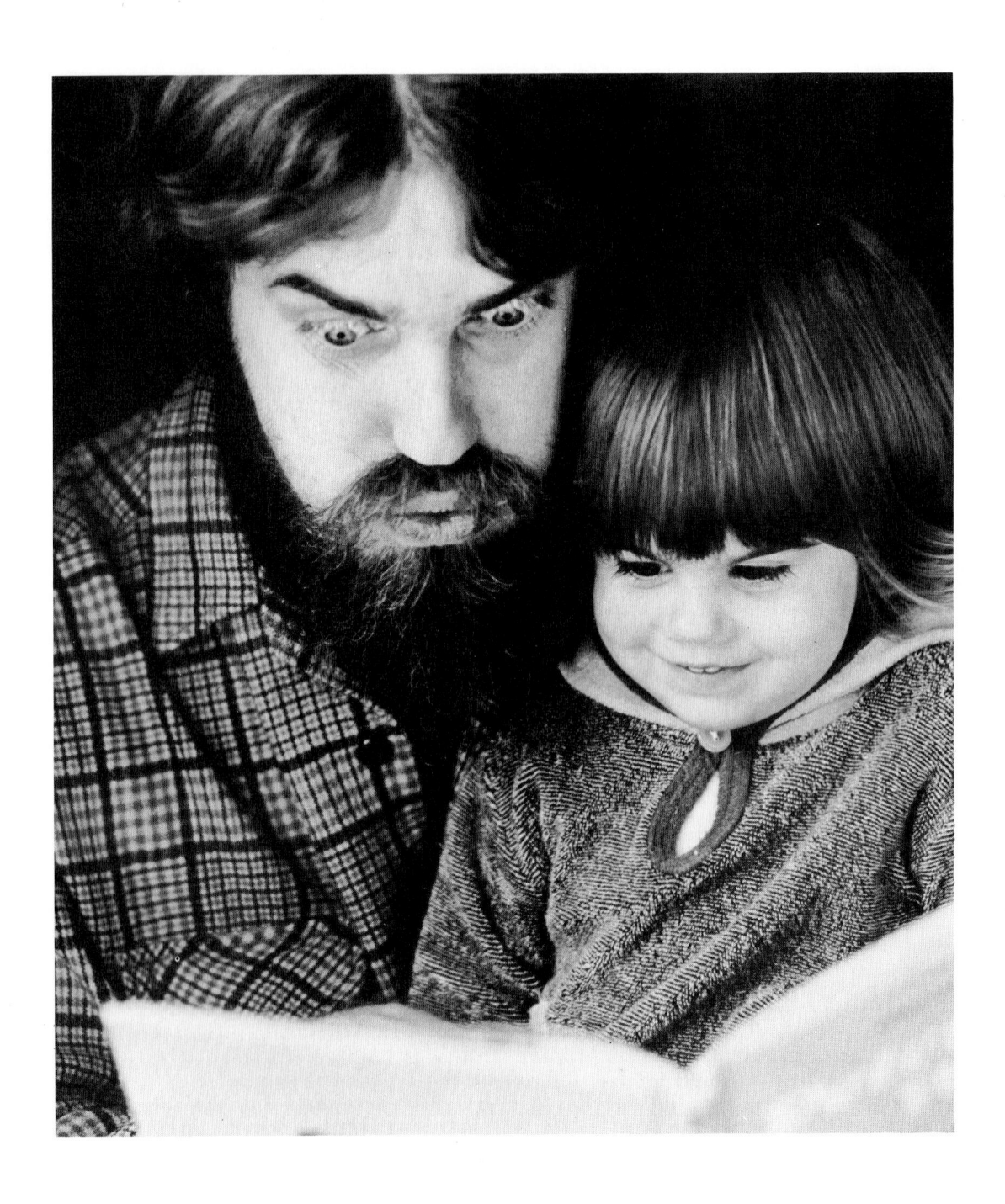

their eyes is very real indeed, someone or something to take into account as the business of the day unfolds. Your son or daughter may conduct actual conversations with "Gerald" or "Sandra," give him or her a personality, and even bring him or her into the family circle. You may have to set an extra place at the dinner table. And watch out! A terrible tragedy may take place when an unknowing visitor ignores or even sits down on the unseen friend.

In the half-magic, half-real world of the child, a friend you can talk to but not see isn't so illogical. After all, adults converse every day with people out of sight on the telephone; on television, they watch the movements and actions of people who aren't really present. The creation of a mythical playmate is one way a child works out the sometimes shifting borders of reality and learns for him- or herself what's real and unreal.

The imaginary playmate also fulfills another role. Your son or daughter didn't spill the milk on the new tablecloth: "Gerald did it." "Sandra," you may be told, "opened the gate," and allowed your three-year-old to escape from the yard. And if you don't buy the story of Gerald as scapegoat, you may hear the child afterward—criticizing Gerald in the same firm tones you used minutes before. Having an imaginary playmate around helps a boy or girl work out his or her own conflicts in a satisfying way. (Sometimes a stuffed toy or the family dog serves the same purpose.)

Because imaginary playmates are normal, parents should not do much about them. If Gerald begins to interfere with family life—if you have to buy an extra ice-cream cone for him, for example—you may have to put your foot down a little and suggest that Gerald come another time. Don't deny that Gerald exists—it's fruitless; his closest friend won't believe it anyway—but don't be caught up in playfully encouraging the fantasy, which will only confuse the child further. As the lyrics suggest in the children's song, *Puff, the Magic Dragon*, one day the playful fantasy will just fade away, and Gerald will disappear from the family circle forever, a welcome visitor for a time whose stay is no longer necessary. You may actually find yourself missing him more than the child does.

STORIES AND STORY TIME

Reading or telling stories to your youngster takes on special significance when he or she is about 2½ and has enough grasp of language to understand more of the tales. The first stories needn't be anything elaborate. In fact, the best ones are those you invent yourself.

A regular story hour is fun for parents, too: There's something enjoyable about snuggling up with a little one and taking him or her (and you too!) into a world of enchantment. A picture book can provide the story or just be a prop: you can point to the pictures and improvise a narrative around them. Remember what you said, though, because your listener will—and will insist that it be told the same way again. Make up stories in which your child is the central figure. And if you're artistic—or even slightly so—you can draw pictures that tell the stories.

The most popular tales among two- and three-year-olds are short on words and long on action. That's why *Mother Goose* has been such a favorite for so many years. Don't just read the stories—act them out. A mommy or daddy who can huff and puff like the Big Bad Wolf or squeal like the Three Little Pigs is the most popular storyteller. Good storytelling for a child also calls for questions, pauses for effect, and reaction from the child. "And what do you think the little pig said then?" brings a delighted, "Not by the hair of my chinny-chin-chin!"

Words to a two-year-old aren't heard just for meaning; they also have rhythm and sound. That's why rhymes are more popular than plain old prose. Read with expression, excitement, and anticipation, and your child will enjoy it most.

AN EAR FOR MUSIC

Between two and three a child begins to like music, too. The child's a little young for Beethoven, Basie, or the Beatles; a simple tune will do. The best ones have a prominent melody and a strong beat. Nursery jingles and marches meet these qualifications—and so, you'll find, do television commercials.

William or Wanda won't yet have perfect pitch. The ability to carry a tune successfully won't develop until about the age of four. But the child will love your singing—however off-key—and probably will plunge in with his or her own little monotone. Children quickly settle on favorites, from lullabies to *She'll Be Comin' Around the Mountain*, and will insist that you provide encore after encore.

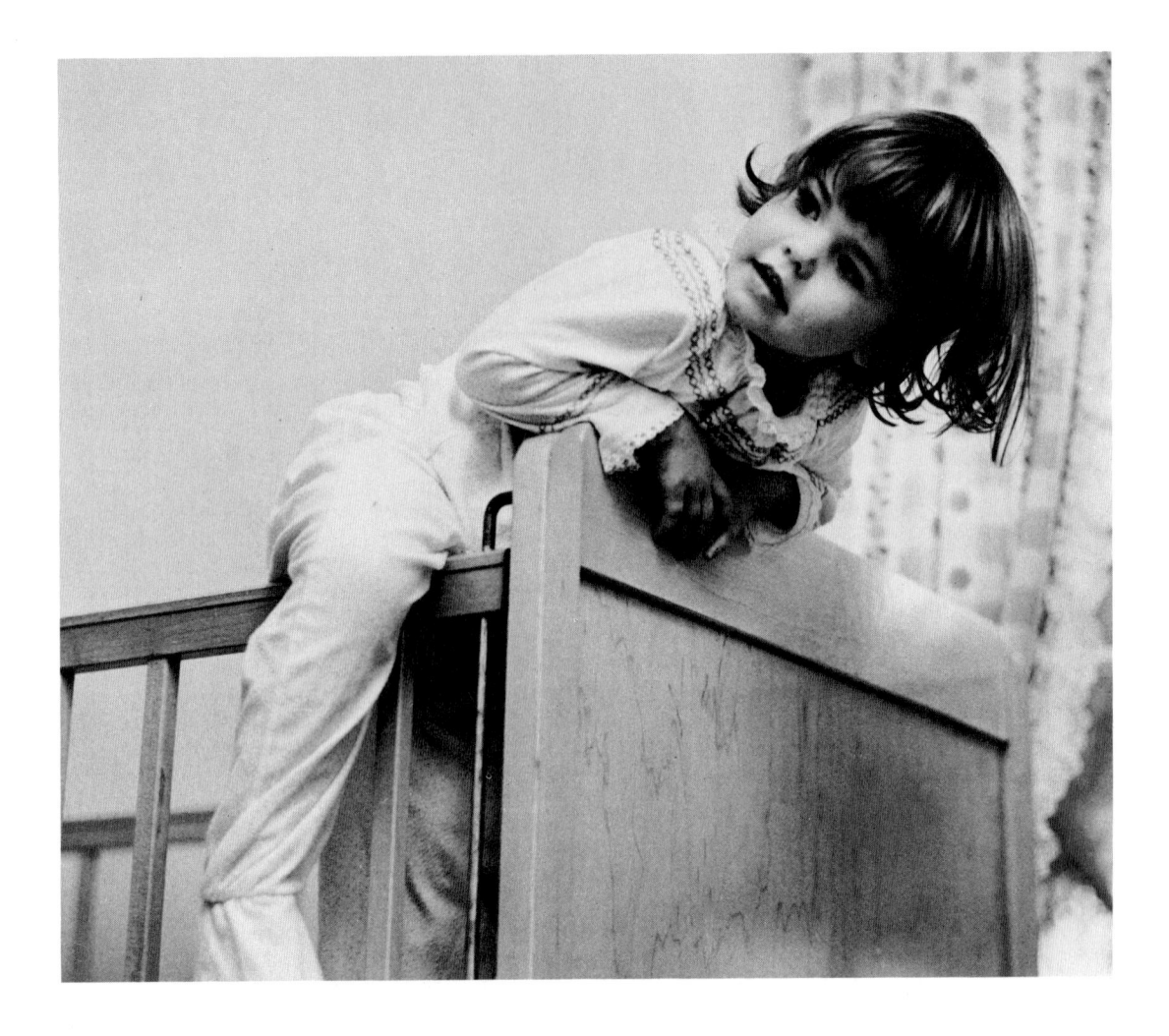

If you can play a guitar or a piano—even if you can only pick out a tune with one finger—your child will be enchanted and, being self-reliant, will want to try it alone. A windup music box that plays a simple tune is a favorite toy for many two-year-olds. A stuffed animal with its own built-in music box is a good, soothing bedtime companion.

Although a two- or three-year-old is too young to manipulate a record or tape player, he or she will enjoy listening to recordings. You can buy many inexpensive children's recordings containing simple melodies, the old nursery rhymes, or dramatized storytelling. You'll often find these at secondhand stores or garage sales.

TELEVISION AND CHILDREN

The images and voices of the television screen capture the attention of even a two-year-old. Studies show that three-year-olds can identify television cartoon jingles before nursery rhymes and that many four-year-olds are glued to the set as much as four hours a day.

Most parents have mixed feelings about television and its influences. There seems to be little support for the belief that a heavy diet of television damages children's eyes or otherwise hurts them physically, but its effects on impressionable minds are continually disputed. Most parents despair about the drumfire commercials with their buy-buy-buy message and the heavy dose of violence that still continues, even on children's programs. And no one likes to see a child passively watching a television screen when there are so many more active and exciting things to do. On the other hand, television has its

Though few children physically outgrow a crib until the age of four, many two-year-olds can escape it with ease, even with the rail raised (at left). Think about a "big bed" and, in the meantime, keep the rail lowered.

positive side. Children do learn from it, as studies have repeatedly demonstrated; some of the most honored programs are aimed at the preschool set. And, however guilty they may feel about it, almost all parents occasionally find the set to be a convenient baby-sitter. It can be a relief to a tired mother or father to plunk a youngster in front of a television, knowing that he or she will be safe from obvious harm.

One extreme way to handle the problem of television is to throw out the set. A better way is to give children some firm rules about what they can watch and when. And these rules should be taught early, when children first become aware of the television set. Here are guidelines to follow:

• Be aware of your own viewing habits. If television is your chief entertainment, it is naive to expect the child to behave differently.

• Monitor what the child watches. Observe the television fare frequently enough to be satisfied that content is suitable. Even familiar shows should be checked periodically, because some of these programs change approach or story line over the years.

• Retain control of the set. That means the on-off switch. *You* decide what the child can watch and how long he or she can watch it. Call a halt when the time comes.

• Consult television schedules or otherwise familiarize yourself with children's programs so you can influence the child's viewing. Don't automatically assume that a "children's show" is something you'd want your child to watch. Don't unthinkingly assume cartoons are children's fare. Many old and new cartoons are heavily laced with violence.

• Discuss the programs as you would a book. Encourage the child to recall them and tell you about them. Studies show that programs are less frightening or confusing to a child if a parent is present to discuss them. In the same way, commercials have less impact if a child can question an adult about them.

• Don't build the child's life around the television. Schedule other pastimes for weekend mornings or late afternoons. A picnic on Saturday morning is a good substitute for television; late afternoon is a good time for the story hour.

A NEW BED, A NEW CHAIR

When to move your child to a standard bed is strictly a matter for personal preference and pocketbook. Few children physically outgrow the crib until they're four years old or more. A restless sleeper probably ought to remain in an enclosed space until he or she settles down. If you put the child to bed at one end of the crib and always find him or her wedged against the other in the morning, wait a bit longer to make the transfer. You'll probably also want to wait until the child is consistently dry at night, usually between 2½ and 3½ years old.

Most children this age can no longer be kept put by plopping them in the crib. An agile two-year-old quickly learns to scramble over the side and escape, and many evenings will be spent putting him or her into bed—and retrieving him or her again and again. Often, the young fugitive also will flee during the night or rise at the gray light of dawn to toddle into your room and wake you. Some desperate parents try to cover the top of the crib with netting, to prevent escape, but most resign themselves and keep the crib rail in a lower position so the acrobat won't be injured crawling over. Pad the floor with pillows, too, to prevent injury.

When picking a new bed, assume, too, the child will topple from it a few times. Choose a model that is close to the floor. It'll take the child several weeks to become accustomed to the unconfined space. In the meantime, tuck in blankets and linens, and line the floor with pillows. Even though the child is usually dry all night, you'll want to place a waterproof pad between mattress and linens. Toilet accidents will continue intermittently for several years. Pick blankets of synthetic fiber: they can be washed easily, and they reduce the possibility of allergic reaction. Also, the child probably is also ready for a pillow at this time.

The baby also may be ready to eat at the table with you—assuming, of course, you cover the table with a plastic cloth. No doubt your youngster has long since outgrown an infant chair, and even a high chair may be confining. You may wish to substitute a booster added to an adult chair, or you may wish to remove the tray of the high chair for easier access to the adult table.

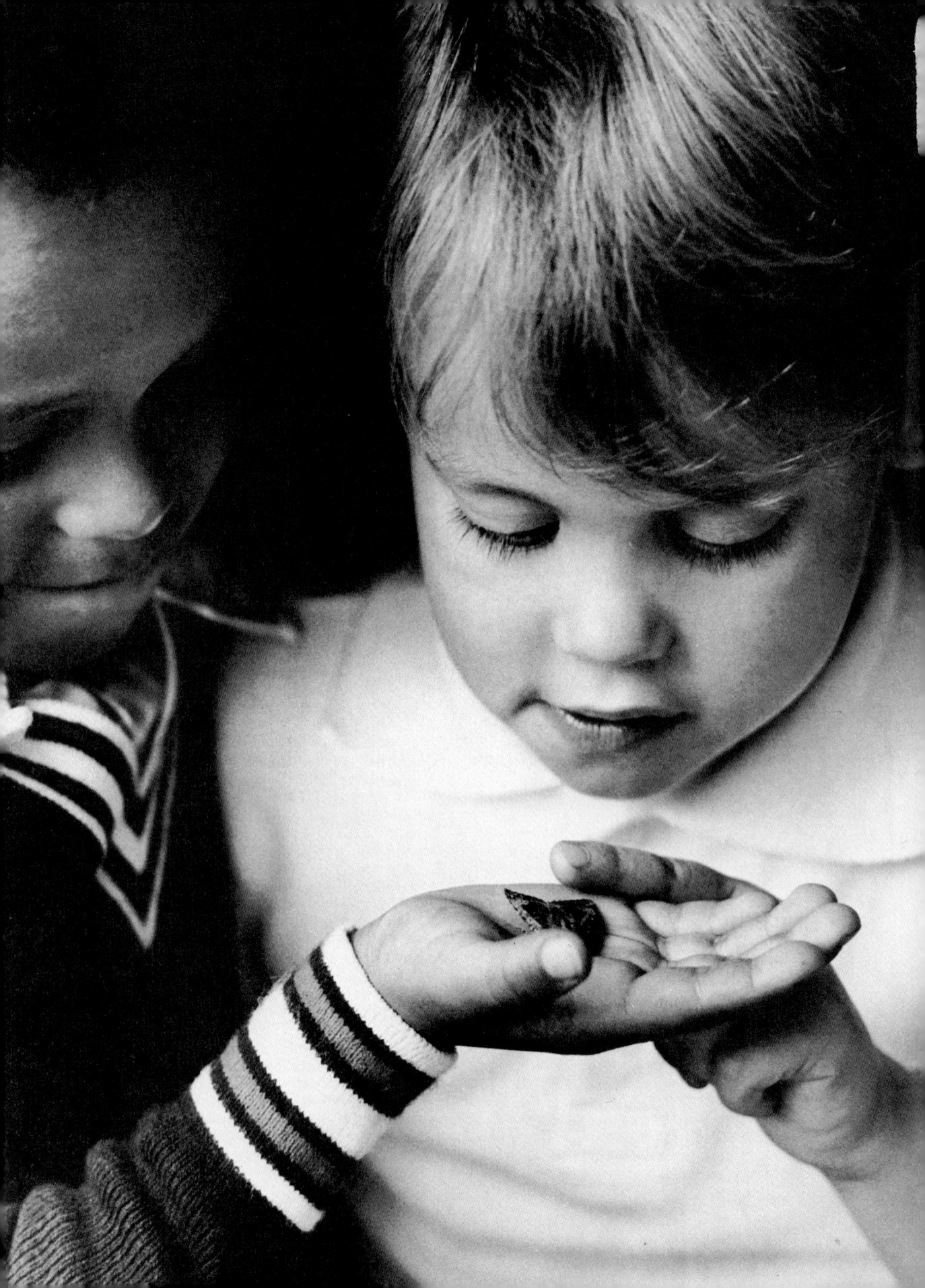

THREE TO FIVE YEARS

HOW THE CHILD GROWS

The average normal four-year-old weighs 37½ pounds and stands 40½ inches, an increase of five pounds and 2½ inches from the year before. The range in size among normal children is 28 to 45 pounds, and 37½ to 43½ inches in height. Usually, girls are smaller than boys, although the height and weight of boys and girls fall within the same range.

Here are some things most normal children may learn to do before the fourth birthday.
• dress without assistance, except for difficult buttons;
• identify colors; make comparisons;
• use plurals and prepositions;
• leave parents easily and play out of their sight for long periods;
• draw a figure recognizable as a human;
• hop on one foot, and maybe skip for a few steps.

At five, an average normal child weighs 42 pounds and is 43½ inches tall. The range of height is 39½ to 46 inches, and the range in weight, 32 to 50 pounds. Here are some achievements of normal five-year-olds;
• define many words;
• catch a bounced ball;
• put on shoes, perhaps even tie them;
• sing a song with a recognizable tune;
• recognize his or her printed name, and perhaps print it.

THE INFANT ADOLESCENT

Between three and five years of age, your son or daughter goes through a transition so profound that it has been called "the adolescence of the preschool years." As in the teens, the person who emerges from this period is quite different from the one who entered it. The three-year-old is still an infant. Your five-year-old is most clearly a child.

Your role changes, too. The three-year-old is increasingly—even demandingly—self-reliant, but many details of caring for the child still fall to you. The five-year-old can dress, eat, go to the toilet, and even bathe with little help from you; sometimes it seems that mother and dad are only called upon to cut meat and deal with difficult buttons. Even social plans may be made without you: Your five-year-old will scurry off to a friend's house unescorted, play out of your sight for long periods, and come and go with minimum supervision. Your child will want it that way, too, and will want a voice in many family plans.

That doesn't mean a five-year-old is a full-fledged adult, even in miniature. The child still lacks judgment. Your guidance is important—essential—to point the child in the right direction and to make decisions that are beyond childish experience. Conversely, you must not expect too much nor push too fast; though no longer a baby, your offspring isn't grown-up by any means.

And the changes don't unfold at the same rate in all children, or even in the same child. A child may quickly mature physically, develop speech slowly, and change emotionally and socially by fits and starts. Your child at five will be different from your child at three, but in retrospect, it may be difficult for you to pinpoint when the transformation took place.

TALK, TALK, TALK

One of the most marked—and most erratic—areas of development is that of speech. Between three and five years of age, most children gradually master the basics of adult communication, and their speech patterns and cadences come to resemble those of grown-ups. But not all children make it over the hurdle at the same pace. Everyone knows an anecdote about a child who spoke only in monosyllables until age three and a half, then blurted out, "Please pass the butter, mother." Your child, though normal, may not have the urge to communicate as quickly as another equally normal child.

The majority of children, however, become increasingly verbal after passing their third birthday. They learn to say just about anything they want to say, and grunts and gestures fade away as a form of communication. Baby talk and mispronunciations continue, but the intricacies of sentence structure and grammar begin to creep in. Gradually, the child peppers conversation with plurals, pronouns, and prepositions. "Me do it" becomes "I'll do it." and "Mommy do it" gives way to "You do it." A four-year-old knows the proper form is "two kitties" and "three puppies" and understands the difference between "under" and "over," "in" and "on." Nearly all normal four-year-olds can define three or four prepositions, according to the Denver Developmental Screening Test, and can deal with such physically descriptive ideas as "cold," "tired," and "hungry." Almost all can give their first and last names.

At the same time, the mind is stretching in other ways, too. Between three and four, your child learns the concept of number, and by the fourth birthday, he or she may be trying to count. The sequence may come out, "1, 3, 7, 2" or "1, 5, 9, 6" for a year or more yet. If you ask the child his or her age, or the number of puppies in the picture, he or she may be able to hold up three or the appropriate number of fingers. At about the age of four, many children learn to recognize their printed name; a few can even laboriously print it themselves, if the name isn't too long and the letters not too difficult. With a pencil and paper, a four-year-old may be able to draw a creditable imitation of a person.

Recognizing colors is another area of progress. Seventy-five percent of four-year-olds can identify basic colors, like "red," "blue," and "yellow," and may even select a "favorite color" (although some children progress more slowly in this area than others). Many have even mastered definitions of words and can identify the opposites of "good," "fast," or "right."

The child's mastery of language may become so complete, in fact, that he or she becomes a nonstop chatterbox, driving parents to distraction with a ceaseless babble that begins at breakfast and continues to bedtime and often beyond; even after the light has been turned out, you may hear him or her in earnest conversation with the teddy bear. Most of this monologue is just practice—the child is displaying a fascination with words and sounds. And these endless, one-sided conversations seldom require acknowledgment or reply. But through your conversation, you can help the child develop language skills, sharpen pronunciation, and learn adult cadences. Continue to talk to him or her, pronouncing words the correct way and using simple but grown-up sentences. Don't overcorrect—but don't use baby talk—and the child will learn the lesson.

"BUT WHY, MOMMY?"

One of the favorite sentences your little talking machine will use consists of three letters: "Why?" You'll hear this inquiry from morning to night, and often after you've responded to one "Why?" you'll hear "Why?" again.

Much of the time the child doesn't really want an answer, just some verbal interaction. He or she is playing with words, testing and examining ideas. Your child likes the attention that comes with your response.

"Why?" also represents a new dimension to a child's ever-growing curiosity. Now he or she has learned there are other ways to make discoveries—tapping the accumulated wisdom of a more experienced mommy or daddy. Your child wants to know what you know and looks to you as a fountain of knowledge.

You don't have to be a walking encyclopedia to deal with these questions, and you don't have to answer them elaborately. Keep your answers simple, with a minimum of details; a child who asks about the man in the moon isn't looking for a lesson in astronomy. Nor do you need to consult reference books or authorities. A few facts are enough.

TOILET ACCIDENTS AND BED-WETTING

Even some time after a child has been successfully urine-trained during the day, accidents will periodically occur. They usually happen because the child is excited, absorbed in play, or in an unfamiliar place and doesn't know the location of the bathroom. Accidents are more frequent when the child is outdoors and hasn't time to hurry home.

Treat incidents like these as casually as you possibly can. Usually, the child is already greatly embarrassed by the whole affair—especially if other children witnessed the event—and no lecture is necessary. Just change the child's clothes, and offer a gentle reminder to start for the bathroom sooner in the future.

When a child has been successfully toilet-trained for a while and then reverts to wetting pants, an emotional cause may be suspected. The arrival of a new baby may cause an older child, especially an only child, to return to babyish behavior long since abandoned. So may a move to a new home. Treat the matter casually, and try to deal with the situation that provoked it; reassure him or her of your love despite the newcomer, or point out that the house is new, but mommy and daddy are still here.

Repeated accidents without an obvious emotional explanation may be caused by an infection or irritation of the urinary tract. Such conditions are more common in girls than in boys; sometimes bubble bath may be the culprit. Consult your pediatrician, who can evaluate the condition and prescribe medication to treat it. A breakdown in toilet training also may be caused by an inborn structural defect in the urinary system. Such conditions can be corrected surgically.

About nine of ten children can remain dry through the night, most of the time, by four years of age. Night training requires much more time than daytime training, however, so don't be surprised if your youngster still has occasional accidents at night until the early school years.

As with daytime toilet accidents, a seemingly spontaneous recurrence of bed-wetting in a child who has been reliably trained to stay dry at night may indicate an emotional or even a physical problem.

As the child nears the fifth birthday, the number of hours spent sleeping at night usually declines to ten or 11. Schedules vary from child to child; watch yours to determine the best one.

THE CHRONIC BED-WETTER

Many people think persistent bed-wetting is rare, but actually it is quite common. One study of 992 Baltimore children showed that between one-fourth and one-third of five-year-olds wet their beds at least once a month; two of three bed-wetters, once a week. Ten percent of seven-year-olds were still not reliably dry, and even one in twenty 12-year-olds wets the bed at least once monthly. Contrary to popular belief, boys and girls were represented in about equal numbers. The problem seemed to run in families.

Why presumably trained children wet their beds on some nights while remaining dry on others annoys parents (and the child, too) and mystifies physicians. The theory that they simply sleep more soundly than the rest of us does not stand up in laboratory tests. A child who suddenly begins to wet the bed after years of being dry may have an emotional problem, but this can be ruled out in the majority of cases. Infection or another physical cause seldom is an explanation, although it should be investigated. And it is not a matter of simply being too lazy to get up and visit the bathroom, as weary parents sometimes allege.

A popular theory today suggests a developmental lag in bladder control. Because the condition runs in families, some physicians suspect an inherited slower maturation of certain nerves. Tests have shown bed-wetters' bladders are of normal size but with a smaller "functional capacity." Even during the day, they visit the bathroom more frequently than other children.

If bed-wetting occurred nightly, it might seem less a problem; constant precautions could be taken. It's the intermittent pattern that causes such friction between child and parent. Repeatedly having to get up in the night to wrestle with wet pajamas and bedsheets leads to the conviction by parents that the child "just isn't trying." It can arouse overwhelming feelings of downright anger, even toward a small child. The first step toward a solution is acknowledging the anger, not trying to make the child feel guilty or ashamed, or calling him or her a "baby," which only complicates things further. Success against bed-wetting can only be achieved by parent and child working together.

Simple measures should be tried first. Place a plastic liner over the mattress and moistureproof sheeting between mattress and linens. Be sure the child visits the bathroom just before retiring. Limiting fluids before bedtime may help, if you don't become so obsessive about it that the child winds up thirsty. Encourage the child to go to the toilet during the night, but it's not necessary to get up with him or her. Install a night-light in the bedroom and bathroom to make night visits easier.

Bladder-training exercises also work for some children, usually those of school age. The child is encouraged to drink large amounts of water during the day, then is urged to wait as long as possible before using the toilet. After a few days, the intervals between visits are said to increase, and within three weeks, according to some reports, children also stay dry at night. Apparently by conditioning the bladder to hold greater volumes during the day, bladder capacity at night is also enlarged.

Your pediatrician may prescribe nightly doses of a medication, imipramine, to control bed-wetting. Imipramine's mechanism of action isn't quite certain, but repeated studies have demonstrated significant elimination or decrease of bed-wetting in a majority of children treated. Unfortunately, many children may resume wetting the bed within a few weeks when the drug is discontinued.

Another treatment the pediatrician may suggest is the use of a bladder-conditioning alarm apparatus. A small metal clip is attached to the child's underpants and connected to a small bell or buzzer, usually worn on the shirt or pajama top. Wetting the underpants completes a circuit, sounds the alarm, and wakes the child. After a few nights, the child begins to wake more quickly after urination begins and gets up and goes to the bathroom. After a few weeks, the bladder is mysteriously conditioned so that urination does not occur at all. The method has been reported to "cure" up to 90 percent of bed-wetters in two to ten weeks, with only a few relapses. The method fails most often when the child does not awaken in spite of the alarm—even when other members of the family hear the noise.

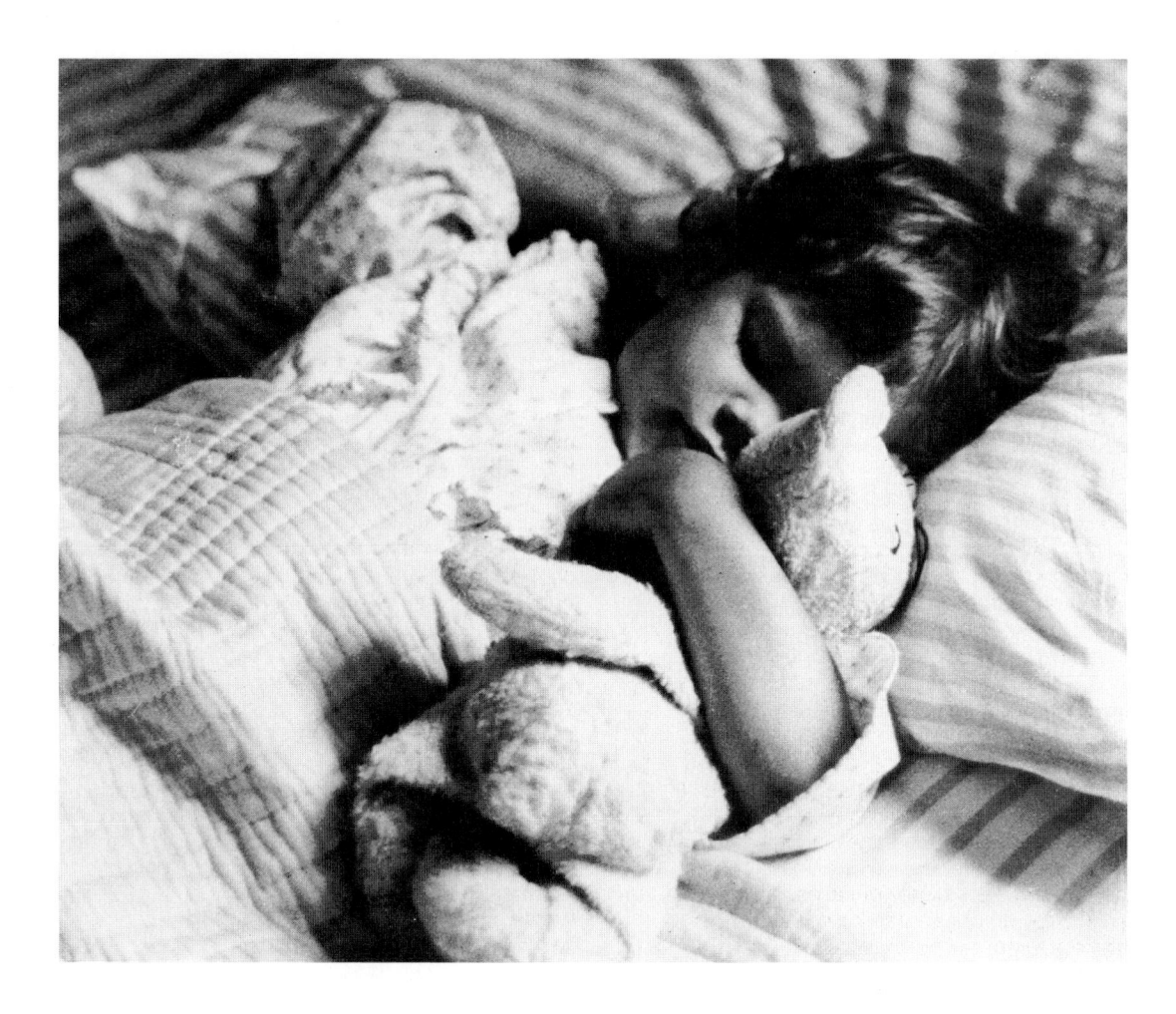

Because the biggest problem—and greatest source of annoyance—is cleaning up, the child usually is willing to take responsibility to offset the parents' natural irritation with the daily hassle. A child old enough to dress and undress can be taught to change nightclothing; if the condition persists to an older age, he or she can learn to change bedding as well. A laundry hamper and linen supply in the room will help.

THE CHANGING SLEEP SCHEDULE

Children usually give up daytime naps around the fourth birthday, although many continue to take a short afternoon nap until they reach kindergarten age. If it continues, the nap may be shortened to an hour and a half.

Some children give up naps gradually. They may discontinue sleeping in the afternoon for a few months, then resume again. Others may lie down each day but sleep only on some occasions and not others. In any case, a four-year-old should continue to have a rest period or quiet time in midafternoon, even if he or she does not sleep. Let the child lie down with a book, pencil and paper, or a quiet toy. An afternoon rest is particularly important if the child is attending nursery school and has a full schedule of activities keeping him or her busy throughout the morning. Even after the nap has been eliminated, insist on a rest period when the child seems overtired or keyed up.

The number of hours spent sleeping at night decreases, too, as the child approaches the fifth birthday. The duration is usually about ten to 11 hours, although the need for sleep varies tremendously. There's no best time for a four-year-old's curfew; it can be determined by family style. A common schedule is bedtime at 8 p.m., with the child arising at 6:30 or 7 in the morning, but this does not have to be rigid. Usually, the later a child retires, the later he or she will sleep. If both parents are working outside the home, you may want to enjoy the child more in the evening and allow him or her to sleep later the next day.

HOW TO PICK A NURSERY SCHOOL

There's no set age for a child to start nursery school, assuming you want to send him or her to one. It depends on the child's temperament, personality, and maturity and your own schedule and resources—plus your need for child-care during the day. The usual beginning is sometime between the third and fourth birthday, although some children start earlier. A child usually attends two or three days a week at first and may gradually work up to a full five-day schedule. A nursery school session normally lasts about two and a half to three hours a day. More and more, nursery school is part of all-day child-care.

When you're trying to decide whether your child is ready for nursery school, here are some questions to ask:

• Is he or she toilet-trained during the day? Many schools insist that the child be out of diapers and know how to use the bathroom without adult assistance. The child also should be able to tell an adult when he or she needs to make a trip to the bathroom.

• Is the child able to take care of him- or herself? In other words, can the child tell an adult when he or she is ill or hurt, get help when needed, and be self-reliant enough to play without constant adult supervision? The child should recognize personal possessions and be able to put on jackets and hats with a minimum of help.

• Does the child leave you easily? Ease of separation doesn't usually come until after the second birthday, unless the child has become accustomed to a preschool or child-care center. Regardless of age, the child often will cling to you during the first visit, and separation throughout the first month may be difficult.

Should your child attend nursery school? There are three main benefits:

• Nursery schools offer encounters and social interaction with peers in a controlled environment. Your son or daughter learns to adapt and accept the rights and demands of other children and to adjust personal wishes to the requirements of the larger group, a socialization process that helps toward molding them into adults.

• The child benefits from the stimulation of early education. Nursery schools don't teach the three "R's," but they do stress learning through personal discovery, and they stress the creativity of arts and handicrafts.

• It's good for parents. Not only does it allow you more time to yourself, even to resume a career, but it offers an opportunity to meet other parents and exchange child-raising experiences.

Nursery schools, like play groups—and like children themselves—come in all shapes, sizes, and pedagogical philosophies. The Montessori schools, for example, stress a structured learning program leading through the entire preschool years. Children start at two to two and a half and advance through methods of personal discovery based on special teaching materials designed by the founder, Maria Montessori. Open schools stress more freedom, with the child able to follow his or her own dictates around a series of "learning centers." Still other nursery schools emphasize arts, language, or crafts.

The best way to discover the best choice of nursery school for your child is to visit several and observe them. Most schools have such days for parents; a few even have one-way glass viewing areas, so you can watch the children without distracting them. Here are things to look for:

Environment. Is the school structurally safe? is the play area well enclosed, preventing easy access to the street? Is there adequate adult supervision to forestall accidents? Is the playground equipment appropriate for children of nursery-school age? Is the school satisfactorily clean by your standards? Are toilet facilities adequate for the number of children? Is medical or nursing help available or on call in case of illness or injury?

Most states or municipalities license or regularly inspect nursery schools, but their minimum standards may not be as high as yours.

Personnel. Do staff members regard themselves as teachers or merely custodians? How does the staff interact with children? Are the children watched or left to their own devices? If a child is hurt, does he or she get immediate attention?

Situation. Are children of similar ages and sizes kept together or are three- and five-year-olds mixed indiscriminately? Some group play is

Should your son or daughter attend nursery school? One advantage is the chance each child has to adapt to other children. The nursery-schooler with a "me-first" attitude quickly learns cooperation is important.

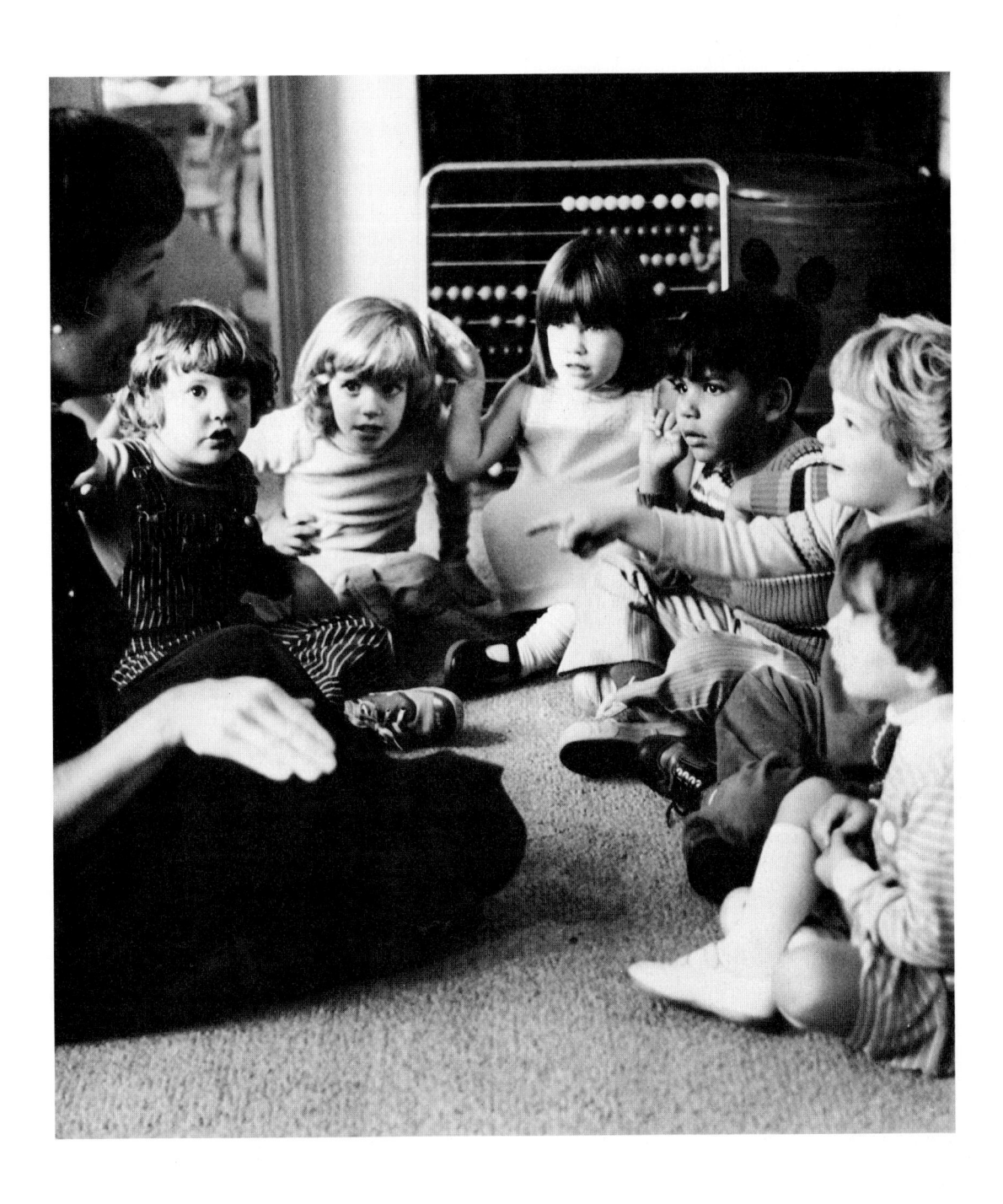

fine on the playground, for instance, but each age group or level of development should have its own time. How is the school structured? Your outgoing child may fit in well at a free-wheeling school, but your shy one may belong elsewhere.

What's expected from you? Many schools operate cooperatively to hold down costs, with one or more parents serving as teachers or teachers' assistants each day. Such economy sounds fine, but you must be sure you have the time to contribute—as well as the desire to do so. Will you have some voice in the decisions of the school—and do you want any—as in a public school, or are the structure and operation unyieldingly the same?

Expenses. Tuition for nursery school ranges widely, and there are no guidelines for what is appropriate. Some hidden expenses, however, may include the distance from school—will you need to drive the child there or take part in a car pool? Is there a bus paid for by the school? Is the school atmosphere rough-and-tumble and the equipment primitive, leading to more wear-and-tear on clothes?

Most educators now agree that children require some form of education prior to beginning formal school (about the sixth birthday). But when that starts and under what circumstances is strictly up to you.

THE MARATHON RUNNY NOSE

To many parents, the years from three to five seem like one continuous runny nose. Nursery school, preschool, or any environment filled with children brings one cold after another. You can expect that a preschool child will have seven to eight colds a year, each lasting about two weeks. The rate is even higher in large families, with each child contributing his or her own breed of viruses.

Apart from passing out handkerchiefs and tissues, there's little you (or your pediatrician) can do to combat a cold. Aspirin or acetaminophen in doses appropriate for the child's age may relieve aches and pains; using a vaporizer at night may make the child's breathing easier. Cough medicines, cough drops, or over-the-counter cold preparations are expensive and their value unproved. A cough syrup made of lemon juice and honey is less expensive, but should not be given to children under one year of age because of the risk that the honey may contain spores that cause infant botulism. The pediatrician may prescribe a decongestant to reduce nasal stuffiness.

Colds are miserable but not life-threatening. You can't do much to help your child avoid them, and maybe you don't want to. Each exposure helps a child build immunity to that particular strain of virus, thus reducing vulnerability later. That's why a child gets so many colds in the first six years of life, when viruses are first encountered, and why the rate of illnesses caused by viruses declines with age.

Most of the time-honored precautions seem to have little effect in preventing a cold; children whose parents observe them faithfully seem to have just as many colds as those whose parents ignore them altogether. Many people believe that drafts, wet feet, and insufficient clothing "cause" a cold, but there is no evidence for this belief. In addition, keeping a child at home to prevent a cold from spreading is unrealistic. Upper respiratory infections are contagious even before symptoms appear.

Be alert, however, for symptoms not normally associated with a cold. Earache, diminished hearing, or swollen glands may indicate a secondary bacterial infection complicating the original viral illness. These infections can have serious consequences, but if detected early, they may be readily subdued with antibiotics. Consult a pediatrician if any of these symptoms accompany or follow a cold. Medical attention should be sought for recurrent or persistent infections that don't subside within a few weeks.

Some parents believe that removing enlarged tonsils and adenoids will help to reduce colds and infections that often follow them, but there is no evidence this is true. Tonsillectomy and adenoidectomy are among the most frequently performed surgical procedures. However, doctors are not even agreed on the value of removing these bits of tissue from the throat and nasal area to relieve the two conditions for which they are most commonly recommended. A tonsillectomy is performed to relieve frequent or chronic infections of the tonsils, usually caused by the streptococcus bacteria; an adenoidectomy to relieve repeated ear infections. Both tissues are known to play a part in the body's defenses against infection, and enlargement of tonsils and adenoids in normal children may indicate these tissues are combating the cold virus, not that they are its victims. As the child grows and the number of infections decreases, the adenoids and tonsils normally shrink in size.

Although enlarged adenoids and tonsils may "squeeze" the eustachian tube connecting ear and throat—thus preventing proper drainage of fluid from the middle ear and increasing chances for infection—additional obstruction may result from slow maturation of the tube itself. If so, it's a problem that cures itself with time. Instead of adenoidectomy, some doctors advocate the insertion of tiny polyethylene tubes in the eardrum, as a means of providing proper drainage from the middle ear.

LYING, STEALING, AND DIRTY WORDS

Not all three- and four-year-olds are angels, and sometimes yours will probably behave in ways you don't approve of.

Falsehoods—you can't really call them lies—are common at this age. Nor can you call them bad—some are so transparent they're funny. A three-year-old still lives in a fantasy world, where impulses and wishes are just as real as facts and deeds. If he or she tells you an elephant ran into the room, upset the milk cup, and raced out again, it's not an attempt to mislead you, nor is it said out of malice. That's what the child wishes were the explanation for the accident. Knowing you may be disappointed or angry, he or she gives you a fabricated account—or more.

Don't engage in a power struggle over an occasional lie. If you accuse the child of lying, his or her instinct is to deny it—and to believe the denial. Show that you disapprove of lying, but use the occasion as an educational experience: "Well, that sounds like a tall story to me," or "I don't care if you broke the cup or Jimmy broke the cup. In this family we don't play with the china." Your answer allows the child to save face, while you get the point across in a fashion that will remembered.

As the child grows older and is better able to distinguish truth from untruth, you can substitute reason. A four-year-old is sensitive to his or her own feelings, as well as those of others, and your talk can be couched in those terms. "I don't like it when you tell fibs to me" lets the child appreciate the consequences of lying in a way he or she can understand.

A five-year-old who lies habitually should cause you to reexamine *your* standards. Children usually tell lies under pressure—when they fear the truth will disappoint you or perhaps cause them to be punished. A five-year-old knows when he or she has failed or fallen short of your expectations. A sustained pattern of lying may indicate that your standards are beyond reach or that you have restricted the child too greatly.

Taking other people's possessions (and, often, lying about it) is another step in growing up. Stealing by a three-year-old is just another manifestation of the child's being dominated by wish and desire. If the child wants something, he or she takes it, because the social limitations adults understand haven't caught up with the child's self-centered impulses. It isn't a serious matter nor is it a precedent. Stealing also may recur at five. At either age, don't ignore the event; just bring it up and deal with it openly and then close the subject.

Don't make a major fuss, and don't directly accuse the child of stealing. If you do, the child may simply deny taking anything at all. "I don't care how it got here. That's Johnny's toy and you take it back" is better than a direct confrontation. "You stole Johnny's toy. I saw you take it" may simply encourage the child to steal more skillfully the next time.

Again, you may wish to examine your own standards. Preschoolers seldom steal because they lack personal possessions or because they are deprived. In fact, their thefts may indicate that you have not conveyed the message that other people's property must be respected.

Even a three-year-old quickly picks up blue language and may repeat it, often under embarrassing circumstances. The words sound so odd coming from a tiny mouth that you may laugh in spite of yourself. That may be the worst thing you can do: Knowing such words are good for a laugh, the child may repeat them again later. Don't ignore the words, either. Just bring the matter to the child's attention by saying that words like these aren't used by anyone in your family and that they shouldn't be used again.

Mischief also becomes part of a preschooler's routine—and a bone of contention with parents. Exasperating as it may be when the child pours salt into the sugar bowl, you can usually endure such incidents. Even a pattern of impishness—hiding Daddy's hat, smearing soap on the bathroom mirror—can be written off to harmless devilment. But if the mischief is consistently damaging or destructive, more serious intervention may be needed. A lasting streak of destruction also may indicate the child is troubled and unhappy; an emotional explanation may be looked for.

MONEY, TOYS, ALLOWANCES

Sometime during the preschool years, a child understands that money has value and can be used to obtain possessions. He or she doesn't know much about it and probably can't distinguish between a penny and a dime. By the age of four, most children know that two coins are more desirable than one coin, but they don't understand much beyond that.

Simultaneously—and with the aid of television advertising—children begin to desire toys or other articles that appear on the screen or are seen in stores. Their desires put parents in a bind. You want to buy things for your child, but your resources are limited, and the child doesn't understand either value or limitations.

You'll find yourself saying "No" a great deal during this period—and you may find it answered with a great deal of protest and rage. It's difficult for a child to comprehend why a toy can be bought one day and not another. You'll just have to be firm, distract the child when you can, and endure the outburst when you can't. You can reason more successfully with a four- or five-year-old. By then, most children have learned they can't have everything, although they may continue to want it. You can sometimes tell them when a gift may be bought—"the next time Mommy and Daddy go to the store"— since their sense of time is still vague. Purchases also can be used as rewards.

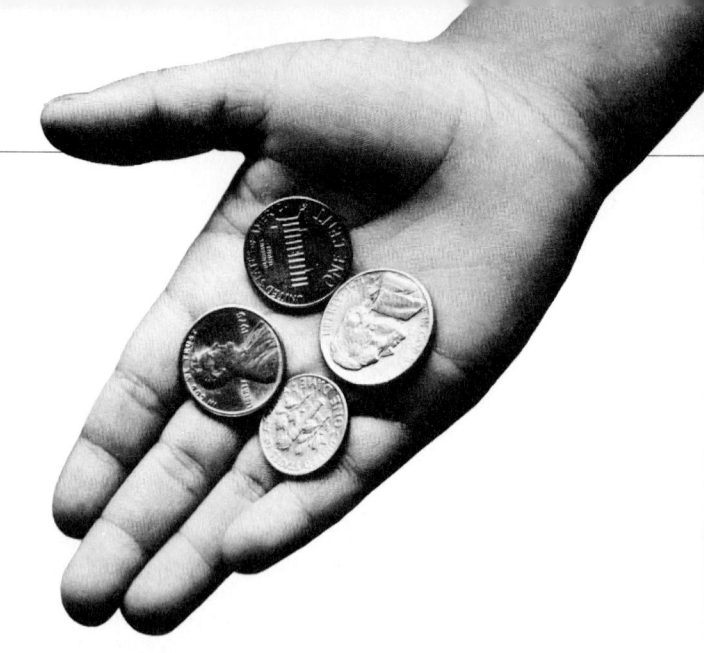

A child hasn't much use for an allowance until the age of five, when it should be given in small amounts but with the provision that the child can spend it as he or she chooses. This gets across the principle of thrift, as well as the idea of deferred gratification.

Some children respond to a special day when they can receive a reward. Saturday can become Candy Day or Treat Day, for instance, with a small budget earmarked for that day. The amount can be based on the child's age, with money subtracted for each time candy is requested in the interim.

MANNERS AND COURTESY

A three-year-old can learn to repeat the words and phrases most of us use in polite discourse, words like "please" and "thank you." No special lessons are involved in the process. If you as parents are courteous in exchanges with others, and especially with each other, the child will quickly pick up those expressions. If you make a game of "please" and "thank you," their use will be habitual by the time the child is old enough to attend school.

In the same way, your courtesy and thoughtfulness with others will be imitated by the child. As he or she grows older, you can expand the lesson by using words, explaining that people are kind and considerate toward one another because they expect the same treatment in return. Explain simply, yet directly, that all of us are interconnected, and if we offend other people, we will lose their love and support.

Despite these lessons, some children act aggressively toward others: A three-year-old may hit, kick, or bite playmates. You can explain that people have other, better ways to express feelings. Anger is normal, you may say, but telling people you're angry is more acceptable than punching. As with many lessons, you can't expect the child to assimilate this stricture in a single setting. You may have to repeat the lesson several times. But remember not to lecture; keep your message short and direct.

What if other children hit your child? Youngsters quickly learn for themselves to deal with an aggressor. Usually, they just give him or her a wide berth; they will say frankly, "I don't want to play with you." This ostracism is often more effective than striking back. With some children, however, it has just the opposite effect: the aggressive child strikes out even more, hoping to gain more attention by doing so.

In such an event, you'll have to teach your child the limits of tolerance. Most of us discourage children from hitting others or striking back when attacked. But if a child allows him- or herself to be bullied repeatedly, the pattern will continue. In this case, you must make it clear to the child that the whole world isn't reasonable; aggressive people must often be dealt with in an aggressive, physical way when they repeatedly overstep the bounds of tolerance.

OBEDIENCE, REWARD, PUNISHMENT

Obviously, you want your child to do what you say when you want it done. Always give directions with confidence they will be carried out. Don't be tentative; be firm in a way that leaves no room for argument or "Why, Daddy?" But don't expect a three-year-old to obey or perform according to your expectations every time.

As your child grows older, you expect that he or she will distinguish approved behavior from the disapproved variety. Approved behavior brings reward and reinforcement; disapproved behavior brings unpleasant consequences. The relationship between behavior and consequences is the basic lesson of discipline. Those consequences must be appropriate to the act and tolerable to both parent and child.

For gaining approved behavior, reward is the best motivator. Of course, every child needs reward, in the form of positive feedback, completely apart from discipline. But rewarding a child—even with something so basic as a hug—is also a teaching technique. That doesn't mean you should give a bribe to produce proper behavior. It does mean you should link the reward directly to the act. Reward should be bestowed for specific acts of behavior a child can understand and should be produced immediately. Asking a four-year-old to be "good" all afternoon in return for a bicycle next Christmas calls for vague behavior and a distant reward. Tell him or her to pick up toys and praise the child afterward—deed and reward are then readily and unmistakably linked.

With older children, reward need not be immediate, but steps toward an eventual reward should be taken at once. Employing a system of delayed reward, you can give the child a penny (or a gold star) for each night he or she remembers to brush the teeth.

For disapproved behavior, you want an act that communicates your displeasure. Just showing by expression or attitude your unhappiness may be enough. "Time out" is another. That means physically separating the child from you and from the scene—banishing him or her to the bedroom, bathroom, or corner. Using a timer with an alarm helps to make the point. Ignoring the child's behavior, surprisingly, also may be effective. When a child persists in an annoying act, even punishment may reinforce the behavior by giving it attention; when mother screams, at least the child is being noticed.

Almost all parents resort to physical punishment occasionally. Spanking works best

Reward is the best answer for good behavior. It needn't be elaborate, so long as the action and reward are linked in the child's mind. Even a simple hug will tell your son or daughter that some ways are better than others.

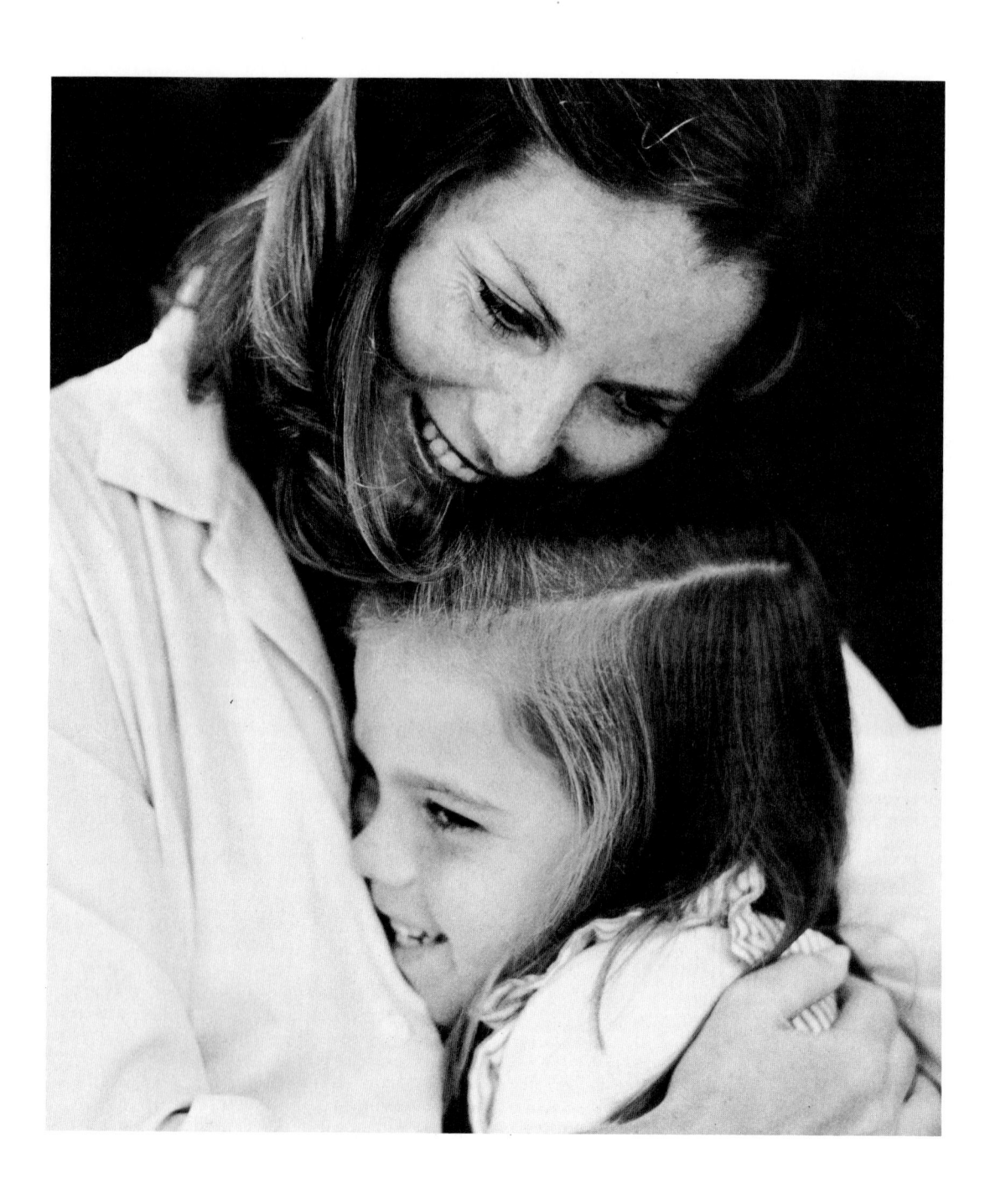

when directly connected to the misdeed and administered immediately. Children can understand a swat delivered in anger better than being deliberately "turned over the knee" for their own good or being punished "after Daddy comes home." By school age, physical punishment is outdated. Being whacked is degrading to a five-year-old.

The least effective motivator is the unfulfilled threat. If you repeatedly tell a child, "Don't do that or I'll spank you," you must be prepared to carry out the punishment if the disapproved behavior continues. Otherwise, the only lesson the child learns is that Mother or Dad talks a lot but doesn't do much.

BUT WILL HE OR SHE OUTGROW IT?

Some behavior that seems attractively cute at three should be worrisome if it still persists at five. A toddler who walks unsteadily is merely amusing, but a hesitant five-year-old may legitimately concern the parents. A three-year-old who calls his sister Barbara "Babawa" gets a laugh; a five-year-old with a lisp may be the target of other children's taunts. Parents may be told (or may tell themselves), "He'll outgrow it." "She'll come around soon." But will he? Will she? When should you be concerned about your child's development?

Physical and behavioral progress covers a wide range, as this book has tried to show. Some problems that worry parents are actually well within the spectrum of normal growth; the child is simply marching to a different drummer, adhering to a personal inner rhythm. Yet early detection of a problem is important. The sooner it's discovered, the more readily it can be corrected.

Obviously, warning signals to parents may differ according to the area of development. But here are general guidelines for intervening in developmental problems that worry you.

• Follow your own instincts. Parents see the child most—and under the greatest variety of circumstances. Don't be swayed by your mother-in-law's diagnosis, "That child walks funny," or, conversely, by a neighbor's judgment, "My sister walked like that, too, and she grew up just fine." (On the other hand, respect the judgment of a trained outsider, a teacher or child-care specialist, for instance, who can professionally compare your child with many others.) If it looks wrong to you, by all means seek help. But don't be goaded just because it seems a child's contemporaries are ahead of him or her.

• Consult your pediatrician, but if you are not satisfied with the verdict, ask for a consultation or seek a second opinion. If you're still concerned, try to identify the leading authority on the problem in your area, and seek his or her advice. But don't shop for doctors, which is expensive and counterproductive, and don't be put off by a doctor's "He'll outgrow it." If you're still worried, ask for any examinations or tests that may clear up the matter once and for all.

• Once the verdict is in, be prepared to deal with it. If examinations show normal bone structure, you can be sure a child will eventually overcome a "funny walk." An exam that shows no structural defect in a lisping child's vocal organs can be similarly reassuring. Be patient in helping the child grow out of the condition. Don't call a stammer or lisp to his or her attention or urge him or her to try to walk differently. Pointing out the problem may only ingrain it more deeply and make it more difficult to overcome.

• Be alert for possible behavioral problems, as well as those of physical development, and seek help if concerned. Most preschoolers lie sometimes, but a chronic liar may require help. Youngsters play with matches, but one who consistently sets fire needs professional assistance.

• Don't worry about minor habits or mannerisms. Preschoolers often develop such habits as nail-biting, face-twitching, stuttering, or stammering. A few may suck their thumbs again after having given up such consolation. The less you say about these conditions the better. Unless such habits are part of a persistent pattern of emotional tension, most of them disappear within a short time.

Ninety-nine out of 100 children outgrow the problems that concern their parents. But if your child does need help, get it as soon as possible.

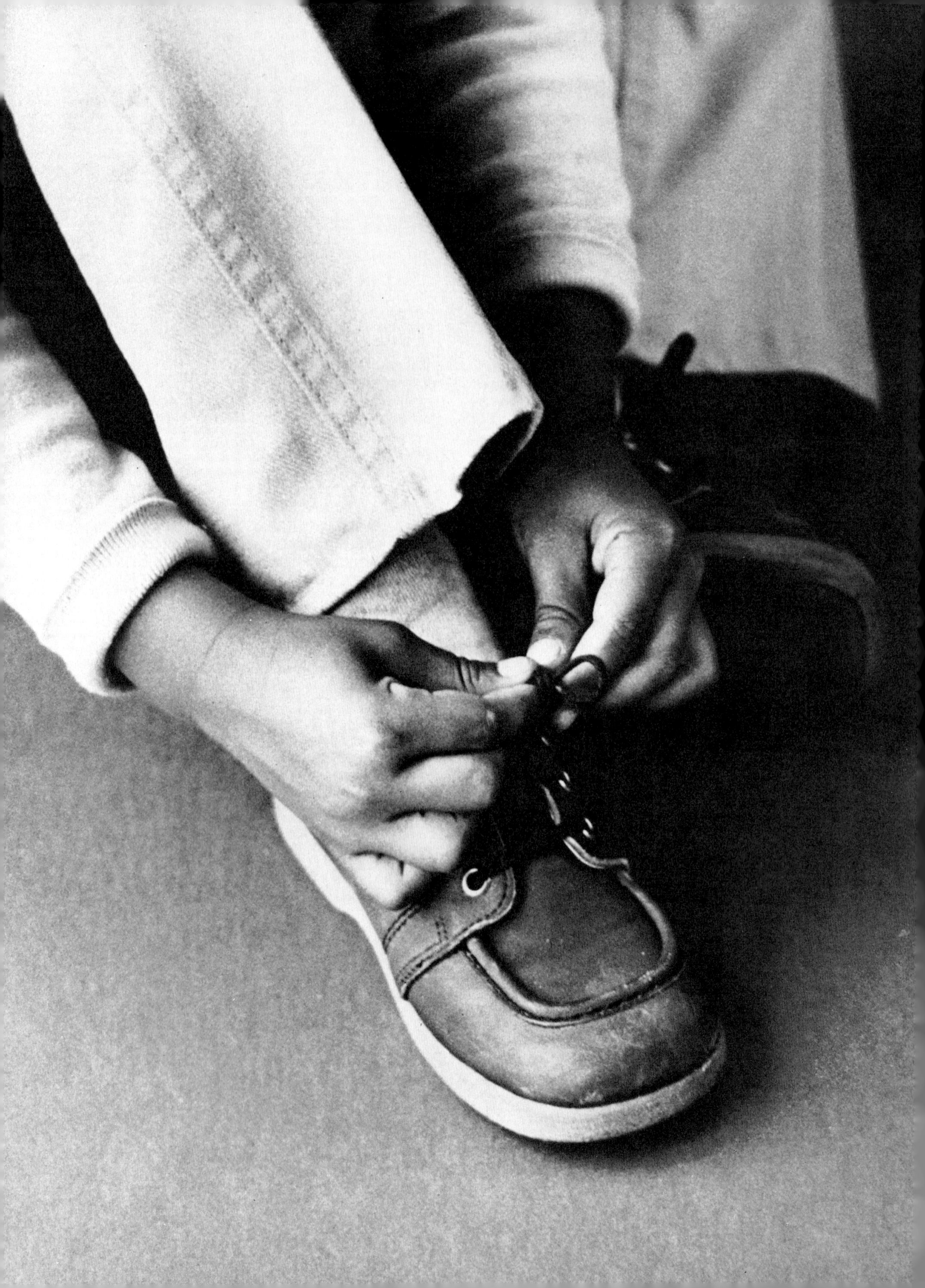

FIVE TO SIX YEARS

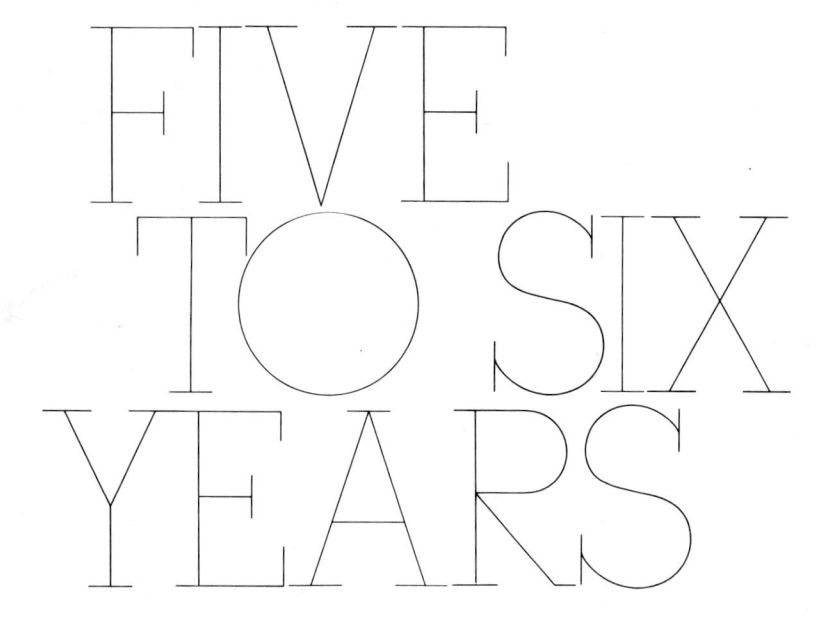

HOW THE CHILD GROWS

Between the fifth and sixth birthdays, the average normal child gains five pounds and grows 2½ to three inches. Average weight is 47 pounds; average height, 45½ inches. The range of normal weight is 35 to 55 pounds; the range of height, 43 to 49 inches.

Between five and six years of age, most children can do the following:
- put on and take off most clothing and probably tie shoes;
- print their first name, if it isn't too long or difficult, and recognize it;
- know both first and last names and be able to tell them to an adult;
- count from one to five in proper sequence and perhaps from one to ten;
- make a recognizable drawing of a person, including arms and legs;
- take care of toilet needs with only very rare accidents;
- wash face and hands and brush teeth with supervision;
- identify most colors;
- understand that a nickel or dime is a more valuable coin than a penny.

A CHANGE IN THE MENU

After several years of picking at food and acting as if eating it were somehow foreign to the laws of human nature, your five-year-old's appetite may suddenly begin to increase—the result of a new upturn in the growth rate.

Over the next three years, the average normal child gains 15 to 20 pounds. The change won't be an abrupt one, however, and you may not immediately notice that your child is eating more until his or her clothes begin to look too small!

Mealtime is now a family occasion, and no special diet is necessary for the growing child. The proper nutritional balance in the food you serve the rest of the family is fine for a five-year-old. He or she will still probably prefer simple food and may reject strongly flavored or heavily seasoned dishes. Most children at this age are still leery of cooked vegetables but will eat raw carrots, celery, cucumbers, and even cauliflower. Fresh fruits provide important nutrients, and most children have several favorites. Fruit juices are popular, too.

By now, your child may have a well-developed taste for sweets and junk foods, and you may want to restrict their consumption.

Milk remains a useful ingredient in a child's diet but need not be consumed in the quantities of the early bone-building years. One or two glasses a day is plenty. Any more only fills up the child and quenches the appetite for other equally useful or even more important nutrients. Skim or fat-free milk is adequate.

You don't have to give your child vitamin tablets if he or she is receiving a balanced diet, although you may wish to continue them. If the local water supply is not fluoridated, fluoride tablets may be continued as well.

A five-year-old's busy social schedule may interfere with regularly scheduled mealtimes; he or she will want to gobble on the run to resume romping with friends. You may feel you almost have to tie the child to the chair to get a decent meal eaten. Later, when everything is put away, the child may return, sniffing for snacks. Maintain your rules of regular mealtimes, but you can allow the child to leave the table as soon as he or she is finished.

THE SCHOOL BELL RINGS

Until now, home and family have been the dominant influences in your child's life. Now you'll share that responsibility with the school. A five-year-old probably will spend half a day in school five days a week.

Traditionally, a child begins kindergarten at five, first grade at six. But those starting dates aren't rigid. The spectrum of development among children is very wide, and some five-year-olds are more prepared for the social and educational experiences of kindergarten than others are. Many teachers strive to give children individual attention to bridge these differences, but this can be a demanding task. In any case, "five years old" is a nebulous term. A child who has just celebrated a fifth birthday is probably quite different from the five-year-old who is a month short of being six.

Most kindergartens now stress preparation for academic work, usually in the form of recognizing letters and preparing for reading. An astute teacher recognizes the children who will respond to such work. Unfortunately, children themselves often feel pressured to keep up with their faster-moving classmates. Despite the teacher's best effort, they may feel they're lagging behind and therefore are failures.

Many educators and psychologists recommend that some children wait a year before starting kindergarten or first grade. They may be urged to spend an additional year in nursery school. Boys, in particular, may be less ready than girls in those skills that are needed for school, and some boys are not ready for kindergarten until the age of six.

When the calendar shows your child is scheduled for school, you may wish to ask yourself these questions:

- Is the child socially mature? Can he or she take care of personal needs? Does your child mix well with other children? Does he or she accept separation from you easily?
- What are the child's strengths and weaknesses? Will he or she flourish best in a structured environment or in a more easy-going one?
- How developed is the child's ability with language? Does he or she talk well and understand most words?

Because sight and sound are at the center of effective learning, the pre-school physical is crucial. Vision must be checked thoroughly. An audiogram (below), which measures hearing ability, also should be part of the examination.

Remember the kindergarten year isn't just an academic period. It's a time of transition, as the child moves from a life in the home to one spent increasingly outside it. You want to make that transition as smooth as possible.

THE PRE-SCHOOL PHYSICAL

Although your child has probably been visiting a pediatrician or well-baby clinic regularly, he or she needs a thorough pediatric examination before starting kindergarten. (Indeed, many school districts require some sort of pre-school physical before the child can begin classes.) Schedule it well before school starts, so any problems can be handled easily.

Because the senses are at the heart of learning, the eyes and ears, in particular, should be tested. Sometimes a slight impairment in vision or hearing isn't noticed by the parents and doesn't make itself evident until the child begins to struggle with classroom work. The pre-school physical examination should be more extensive than just measuring the child's ability to read the eye chart posted on the doctor's wall. The doctor should, in addition, check the ability of the child's eyes to focus and, at the same time, look into the possibility of eye infections.

The hearing test should include an audiogram, which measures sensitivity to tones and frequencies as well as loudness. The doctor also should look for accumulated fluid in the middle ear, which can cause mild to moderate hearing loss.

Most doctors want to hear the child speak, too. In case of a "cute" speech pattern, the doctor may recommend the child visit a clinic or speech pathologist, because a speech impairment can hinder proper pronunciation and stand in the way of learning.

At this point, you'll also want to check the child's shots. DPT and polio boosters are due between the fourth and sixth birthdays. In many states, beginning students must produce a complete record of immunizations showing they've received all the recommended shots before they can be admitted to school.

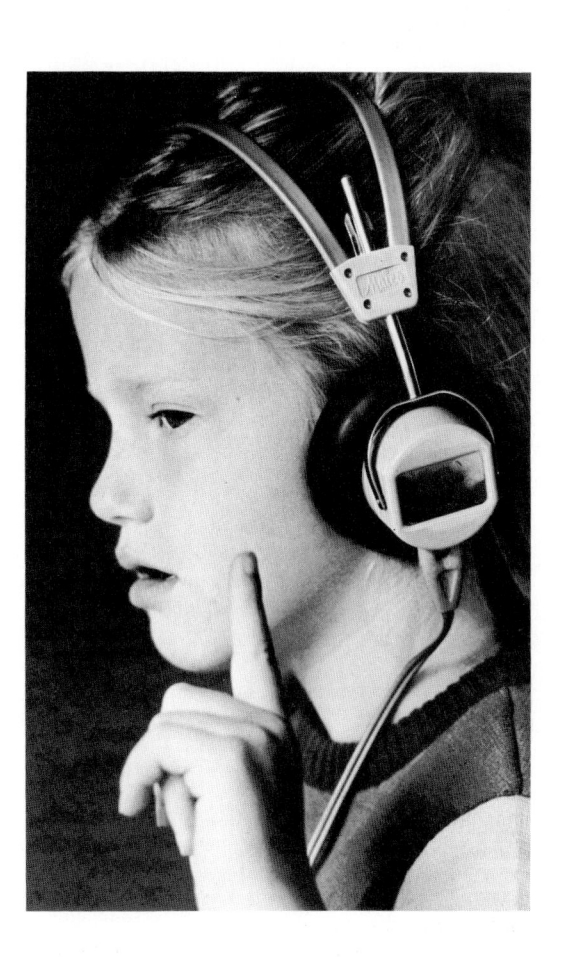

SAFETY ALONG THE WAY

Safety should be the first lesson of kindergarten. If your child walks to school, be sure to cover the route with him or her beforehand. You want a five-year-old to be familiar with the route before trying it alone. If possible, escort your son or daughter to school the first few days and meet him or her for the trip home. If an older child in the neighborhood also attends the school, ask if they can walk together.

Teach the child to observe all the basic rules of pedestrian safety; stop at intersections, look both ways before crossing, and always walk within crosswalks. Teach your child always to stay on sidewalks and to follow the directions given by crossing guards or police who may be on the scene. Also, every child should be taught to walk through an intersection and not run across the street.

A child who rides a bus to school should learn the correct way to enter and leave the vehicle. Even if the driver escorts the child across the street after disembarking, he or she should learn to look both directions before crossing. Go with the child to the bus stop the first few days, and meet him or her on the return trip, especially if the walk home covers several blocks.

School bus drivers usually control children's behavior on the bus. But tell your child to take a seat quietly, to remain in the seat throughout the ride, and not to engage in horseplay while the bus is moving.

Before joining a car pool to transport children to school, make sure that all the parents involved agree on safety regulations. Each car in the pool should have a seat belt or restraining harness for every child; belts or harnesses should not be shared. There should be no more passengers than can be seated comfortably. Children should always enter and leave the vehicle from the curb side, never the street side, and the driver or another adult should help them from the car. At the school, load cars off the street or when a teacher or other school employee is present.

A FEELING OF SECURITY

A five-year-old usually knows his or her first and last name and can recite each of them plainly enough for an adult to understand. The child can usually also print at least his or her first name and probably can recognize his or her name if printed in block letters on paper or on the inside of clothing or boots. Before the first day at kindergarten, help your son or daughter to memorize the family phone number and your street address (or be able to describe the home), so that he or she can tell another adult when lost.

Especially in these days when many parents work or are busy with other duties during the day, schools usually require that you list the name of a friend, neighbor, or relative to be contacted in the event of an emergency when you cannot be reached. The name of the family physician or the child's pediatrician and the work telephone number of one or both parents usually also must be kept on file. However, the child also should be instructed whom to call in an emergency when you are not at home. He or she should know the phone number and address of that person (a neighbor or close relative, perhaps) and how to reach the person's home.

Always instruct the child beforehand in case the routine varies. If he or she is to go to a different home after school, make sure the plan is clear to the child before the school day begins. Many schools require that you file a written note in case of change of plans or, at least, call the child's teacher. If you're not going to be there when the child usually comes home and another person will be waiting, make sure the child expects that. Never let a five-year-old come home to an empty house—it's a scary feeling.

Mark all of the child's belongings, including jackets, hats, and overshoes, so he or she can recognize and find them easily. Try to choose garments that can easily be distinguished, even by a child who is not yet able to read a printed name. Color-code shoes and boots with green (right) and red (left) markers, so he or she can easily match the right piece of footwear to the appropriate foot. You can use a similar color key on gloves and mittens.

THE PARENTS' ROLE

You have a part to play in the child's schooling, too. Even a kindergartener brings home a blizzard of papers and handicrafts for you to inspect and admire. It might be difficult for a busy parent to review every last scrap of paper that arrives, but as often as possible, you should look at the child's work and examine it.

Always find something to praise in the child's work, however difficult it may be to decipher. The leading statement, "Tell me about your picture," is more encouraging to a fledgling artist than an incredulous, "What is that?" Avoid criticism, even constructive criticism, and try not to show amusement at the child's efforts. Laughing at him or her only makes a child feel foolish. Don't overdo the praise, though; even a child recognizes that you can say only so much about a page of printed "b's" and "d's." Try to be specific in your praise. "That's a nice tree" tells the child you really are paying attention.

Like adults, children don't always want to talk about the day's events. Don't pressure with "What did you learn today?" Just show interest and let them volunteer their recital of kindergarten happenings.

Remember that education isn't something that goes on only within school walls. Review lessons as asked by the teacher, but also help the child to review and practice what is being learned. Supply pencils and paper for printing and drawing, for example, and keep a well-stocked library of books that will help him or her reinforce reading techniques. Experiences, visits, and travel also stimulate the child's curiosity and help with informal learning.

Whether or not you join a parents' group at the child's school is strictly up to you; don't be stampeded into membership if you don't feel you have time to devote to it. But visit the classroom when possible, and discuss the child's progress with the teacher. And if you are not satisfied with the teacher or with the school program, make your opinions known.

A SENSIBLE SCHEDULE

Beginning kindergarten may dominate a child's life but shouldn't be allowed to disrupt it. A five-year-old still needs adequate rest, regular mealtimes, and a schedule that keeps activities in perspective.

The need for sleep is gradually lessening, but for most children it remains at about ten hours a night. Because school hours are consistent, bedtime should come at a fairly regular hour, too. Usually, a five-year-old should be in bed by 8:30 p.m. and awaken about 7 a.m. A kindergartener on an afternoon schedule might sleep later. The morning timetable should allow enough time for the child to eat a good breakfast before school begins.

For afternoon kindergarteners, call the child in from play sufficiently ahead of time to allow a brief rest period before school. When the child returns from school, he or she should have another period to rest and unwind, much the way an adult wants to unwind after a day at work.

Entry into kindergarten often is the signal for a flurry of other activities outside the home. Many five-year-olds are enrolled in crafts classes, gymnastics, music lessons, or swimming. These activities stimulate a child and expand his or her horizons but shouldn't be allowed to overwhelm the day. Two regular activities outside the home in addition to school are probably plenty for most children in kindergarten.

BACK TO BABYHOOD

In the first days of school, you may be dismayed to find the child returning to habits that had been given up a long time ago. A five-year-old who has long since stopped thumb-sucking may suddenly pop the thumb back into the mouth; another child may dig out the disreputable "blanky" that provided solace in infancy. Whining and crankiness are common. Some children begin to have toilet accidents or wet the bed after years of being dry and toilet-trained.

These reversals are natural, temporary, and seldom related to specific events at school. Although kindergarten is usually a low-key environment, it's a new and often demanding experience for a five-year-old and quite a step up from nursery school. Youngsters themselves seem to recognize they are moving into an adult world. Although they respond to this challenge, often with eagerness, they also feel pressure that makes them—just as adults do sometimes—long for easier days.

Most children adjust to the new way of life within a few weeks. Because the change in temperament may partially be related to fatigue, you may wish to suggest that the child resume a short afternoon nap for a while. A brief quiet time after the child returns from school also may help. Of course, if the behavior persists or seems to be part of a broader pattern of emotional upset, you should seek assistance.

BACK TO WORK FOR MOTHER?

The majority of women who have worked before pregnancy return to their jobs within six months after birth, according to surveys. But many women prefer to wait until the youngest child enters school before resuming the careers or education that has been placed on hold. If this is your choice, it calls for some shifting of responsibilities for the child who has previously been cared for exclusively by mother at home.

The change isn't always easy for either parents or youngsters. Many children are unhappy to learn that mother will no longer welcome them after school. "How come you have to go to work?" may be a difficult question to answer. Try to explain that although mother likes being at home, she also likes her career or schooling, just as children love their homes but have interests elsewhere. Financial reasons may persuade older children. They can understand that mother's job may enable the entire family to live more comfortably.

Any new arrangement should become a family project. Most fathers today share in child-care responsibilities, but with mother's return to work, fathers may have to take on additional duties. (Some may even choose to become full-time homemakers themselves.) Even young children can take a role. A five-year-old can help to keep his or her own room neat and perform regular chores such as sweeping porches, helping with yardwork, and caring for pets. Older ones can have greater responsibilities.

It's better to establish a regular child-care arrangement outside the home than set up a makeshift one or allow the child to arrive at an empty house to wait. Often, you'll find other parents in the same boat, and a cooperative child-care arrangement can be established.

Other possibilities to be explored include a child-care arrangement at your place of employment, now offered by an increasing number of employers. Sometimes municipalities or schools offer after-school care programs or playground activities that continue until parents finish work. You may be able to find a friend who will supervise the child during the after-school hours.

Whatever course you choose, always be sure school authorities have a phone number of a friend or relative and a telephone number where you can be reached. Discuss with your employer beforehand how you'll handle an emergency.

THE CHILD IS INDEPENDENT

More and more your child is becoming a little adult. Usually able to dial the telephone and self-reliant enough to walk to a friend's home, your son or daughter will make his or her own social plans that must be fitted into those of the rest of the family. In fact, sometimes you'll have that "empty-nest" feeling, as the child spends less time with you and more with peers. It won't be quite so easy to engage in a spontaneous family outing; the child's plans may conflict with yours.

You'll also find that even a five-year-old wants some voice in his or her life. You can't just pick out clothing for the day and expect the child to wear it docilely. Children begin to show tastes of their own—which may clash with yours—and to be adamant about them. Peer pressure and television commercials also shape their ideas.

You don't have to cater to a child's every whim, but you'll have to be prepared to take them into account. You can allow latitude in picking (or buying) clothes by narrowing the selection of shirts, for example, to three and allowing the child to make the final choice of which to wear or buy. The child can follow his or her own social schedule when it doesn't conflict with the family's plans; his or her ideas should be considered but not allowed to sway the family's decision.

You're entering a stage where you'll have to be prepared to say "No" and be unpopular. Although your child is entering a new phase of maturity, supervision still lies with you.

MEDICAL RECORDS

In our mobile society, it's important for you, as well as your physician, to keep family health records. If you move to another town, change doctors, or transfer to a different school, these records you keep can be important references and can be used for consultation.

The examples below will give you an idea of the records you may want to keep. Use them to devise your own, and, when possible, have your physician make the entries personally. If this cannot be done, enter the necessary information yourself immediately after the illness or health event.

This information can then be shown on request to another doctor or to authorities at your child's school. Such information should always be kept up-to-date. You may also wish to file copies of birth certificates, records of inoculation, or other important documents in this part of the book. If you did not receive this information at the time, you should obtain it now to keep your records complete and current.

FAMILY MEDICAL HISTORY

	Birth date	Illnesses
Father	_____	_____
Mother	_____	_____
Brothers	_____	_____
	_____	_____
	_____	_____
Sisters	_____	_____
	_____	_____
	_____	_____

Family illnesses, allergies, or chronic conditions _____

BIRTH RECORD

Date of birth _____
Duration of pregnancy _____
Mother's health during pregnancy:
　Illnesses _____
　Drugs/medications used _____
　Problems _____
Delivery:
　Normal ___ Cesarean section ___
　Medications during labor _____
　Monitoring _____
　Problems _____

Birth measurements:
　Weight _____
　Length _____
Conditions at birth: _____

Type of feeding:
　Breast ___ Bottle ___
Duration of hospital stay (days) ___
Blood type and Rh _____
Other information _____

IMMUNIZATION RECORD

Immunization	Date	Dose	Physician
DPT			
DT booster			
Tetanus booster			
Polio			
Measles			
Rubella			
Mumps			
Tuberculin test			
Others			

ILLNESS & INJURY RECORD

Illnesses:
Nature	Date	Physician

Injuries:

HOSPITALIZATION RECORD

Nature	Date	Physician

Allergies:
_____
_____
_____

Other Information:
_____
_____
_____

DENTAL RECORD

UPPER TEETH
5 4 3 2 1 1 2 3 4 5
1 central incisor
2 lateral incisor
3 cuspid
4 first molar
5 second molar

LOWER TEETH
5 4 3 2 1 1 2 3 4 5
1 central incisor
2 lateral incisor
3 cuspid
4 first molar
5 second molar

AGE TEETH APPEARED

	Upper Teeth		Lower Teeth	
	Right	Left	Right	Left
1	___	___	___	___
2	___	___	___	___
3	___	___	___	___
4	___	___	___	___
5	___	___	___	___

Age

Thumb-sucking _____
Pacifier _____
First brushed teeth _____
Brushed teeth unassisted _____
First flossed teeth _____
First visit to dentist _____
Preventive care _____
Orthodontic procedure _____
X rays _____

45

1 TO 2 YEARS

GROWTH

	Pounds/Ounces
At 18 months	_____ _____
At two years	_____ _____

DEVELOPMENT

	Months
15 months: Use a spoon and spill only a little	_____
Imitate a parent doing housework	_____
Scribble with a crayon	_____
18 months: Remove some or all of clothes	_____
Build a four-cube tower	_____
Walk up steps, holding rail	_____
Point to a baby's picture in a book	_____
Use name for him- or herself	_____
Two years: Combine words to make simple statements	_____
Identify one or more parts of the body	_____
Follow simple directions—if only a single step is involved	_____
Wash and dry hands, with parental supervision	_____
Identify pictures of animals by name	_____
Pedal a tricycle; propel a kiddie car with feet	_____

2 TO 3 YEARS

GROWTH

	Pounds/Ounces
At 2½ years	_____ _____
At three years	_____ _____

DEVELOPMENT

	Months
Dress with supervision and button some buttons	_____
Play interactive games, tag, for instance	_____
Tell first and last names	_____
Use plurals, pronouns, and prepositions in speech	_____
Copy a circle with a crayon	_____
Understand such words as "cold," "tired," "hungry"	_____
Know where things belong and help to put them there	_____
Follow simple, one-step directions	_____
Feed him- or herself almost completely	_____
Be toilet-trained during the day and remain dry all night some of the time	_____
Recognize and identify some colors	_____

3 TO 4 YEARS

GROWTH

	Pounds/Ounces
At 3½ years	_____ _____
At four years	_____ _____

DEVELOPMENT

	Months
Dress without assistance, except for difficult buttons	_____
Identify colors; make comparisons	_____
Use plurals and prepositions	_____
Leave parents easily and play out of their sight for long periods	_____
Draw a figure recognizable as a human	_____
Hop on one foot, and maybe skip for a few steps	_____

4 TO 5 YEARS

GROWTH
Height/Weight

At 4½ years _____ _____
At five years _____ _____

DEVELOPMENT
Months

Define many words _____
Catch a bounced ball _____
Put on shoes, perhaps even tie them _____
Sing a song with a recognizable tune _____
Recognize his or her printed name, and perhaps print it _____
Balance on one foot for ten seconds at a time _____
Walk with a motion from heel to toe _____

5 TO 6 YEARS

GROWTH
Height/Weight

At 5½ years _____ _____
At six years _____ _____

DEVELOPMENT
Months

Put on and take off most clothing and probably tie shoes _____
Print first name, if it isn't too long or difficult, and recognize it _____
Know both first and last names and be able to tell them to an adult _____
Count from one to five in proper sequence and perhaps from one to ten _____
Make a recognizable drawing of a person, including arms and legs _____
Take care of toilet needs with only very rare accidents _____
Wash face and hands and brush teeth with supervision _____
Identify most colors _____
Understand that a nickel or dime is more valuable than a penny

6 TO 7 YEARS

GROWTH
Height/Weight

At 6½ years _____ _____
At seven years _____ _____

DEVELOPMENT
Months

Take care of nearly all personal needs, including bathing, dressing, and going to bed _____
Define many simple words and explain simple concepts
Recognize most letters of the alphabet, perhaps recite them in sequence, and recognize some simple words _____

47

INDEX

A–M

Adenoidectomy, 32–33
Aggressive behavior, 7–8, 35
Allowances, 34
Bed, standard, move to, 23
Bed-wetting, 27–29
Behavior
    aggressive, 7–8, 35
    approved, reward for, 35
    disapproved, 33–34
        punishment for, 35, 37
    problem, 37
    reversals in, 43–44
    two-year-old's, 16
Car pool safety, 42
Chair for eating at table, 23
Clothing, putting on, 8, 16
Colds, 32
Communication
    courteous, 34–35
    dirty words, 34
    second year, 6
    three to five years, 26–27
Courtesy, 34–35
Crib vs. standard bed, 23
Dental care, 10
Developmental problems, 37
Development and growth. See
    Growth and development
Diet
    for five-year-old, 40
    in second year, 10–11
Dirty words, 34
Discipline, 35, 37
Diseases, 32–33
Dressing, 8, 16
Eating
    by five-year-old, 40
    problems in second
        year, 10–11
    self-reliance in, 16
Examination, preschool, 41
Favorite parents, 18
Feeding
    of five-year-old, 40
    problems in second
        year, 10–11
    self-reliance in, 16
Furniture, child's, 23
Growth and development, 46–47
    1–2 years, 5, 46
    2–3 years, 15, 46
    3–5 years, 25, 46–47
    5–6 years, 39, 47
Hands, washing and drying, 8
Health
    illnesses, 32–33
    records, 45
Height and weight. See Growth
    and development
Illnesses, 32–33
Imaginary playmates, 19, 21
Independence, increased, 16, 44
Kindergarten
    and behavioral changes, 43–44
    parents' role in, 42–43
    physical before, 41
    readiness for, 40–41
    safety en route to, 41–42
    and schedule for child, 43
    and security measures, 42
Language
    courteous, 34–35
    second year, 6
    three to five years, 26–27
Lying, 33
Manners, 34–35
Mealtimes
    for five-year-old, 40
    problems in second year, 10
    self-reliance at, 16
Medical records, 45
Mischief, 34
Money, concept of, 34
Music, 21–22

N–Z

Naps, 29
Nightmares and night fears, 18
Nose, runny, 32
Number, concept of, 26
Nursery school, 30–32
Nutrition
    for five-year-old, 40
    in second year, 10–11
Obedience, 35
Order, sense of, acquiring, 8
Outdoor play, 6–7
Parents
    of aggressive children, 7–8
    favorite, 18
    mother's return to work, 44
    schooling, role in, 42–43
Passive vocabulary, 6
Physical, preschool, 41
Play, outdoor, 6–7
Play equipment, 7
Play groups, 19
Playmates, 7–8, 19
    imaginary, 19, 21
Potty training, 11, 13
Preschool physical, 41
Punishment, 35, 37
Records
    growth and development, 46–47
    medical, 45
Rest period, afternoon, 29
Reward, 35
Rituals, 18
Runny nose, 32
Safety on way to school, 41–42
Schedule
    for kindergarten child, 43
    sleep, changing, 29
School
    nursery, 30–32
    See also Kindergarten
School bus safety, 42
Security for kindergartner, 42
Self-reliance, 16, 44
Sleep patterns
    for kindergarten child, 43
    nightmares and night
        fears, 18
    schedule, changing, 29
Speech
    courteous, 34–35
    dirty words, 34
    second year, 6
    three to five years, 26–27
Stealing, 33–34
Stories and story time, 21
Sweets, 10–11
Talking
    courteously, 34–35
    dirty words, 34
    second year, 6
    three to five years, 26–27
Teeth, care of, 10
Television, 22–23
Toilet training, 11, 13
    accidents, 13, 27–29
Tonsillectomy, 32–33
Toys
    desire for, 34
    outdoor, 7
Urine training, 11, 13
    and accidents, 13, 27–29
Vocabulary, 6
Washing and drying of hands, 8
Weight and height. See Growth
    and development
Wetting accidents, 13, 27–29
"Why?" questions, 27
Words, use of
    courteous, 34–35
    dirty, 34
    second year, 6
    three to five years, 26–27
Work, mother's return to, 44

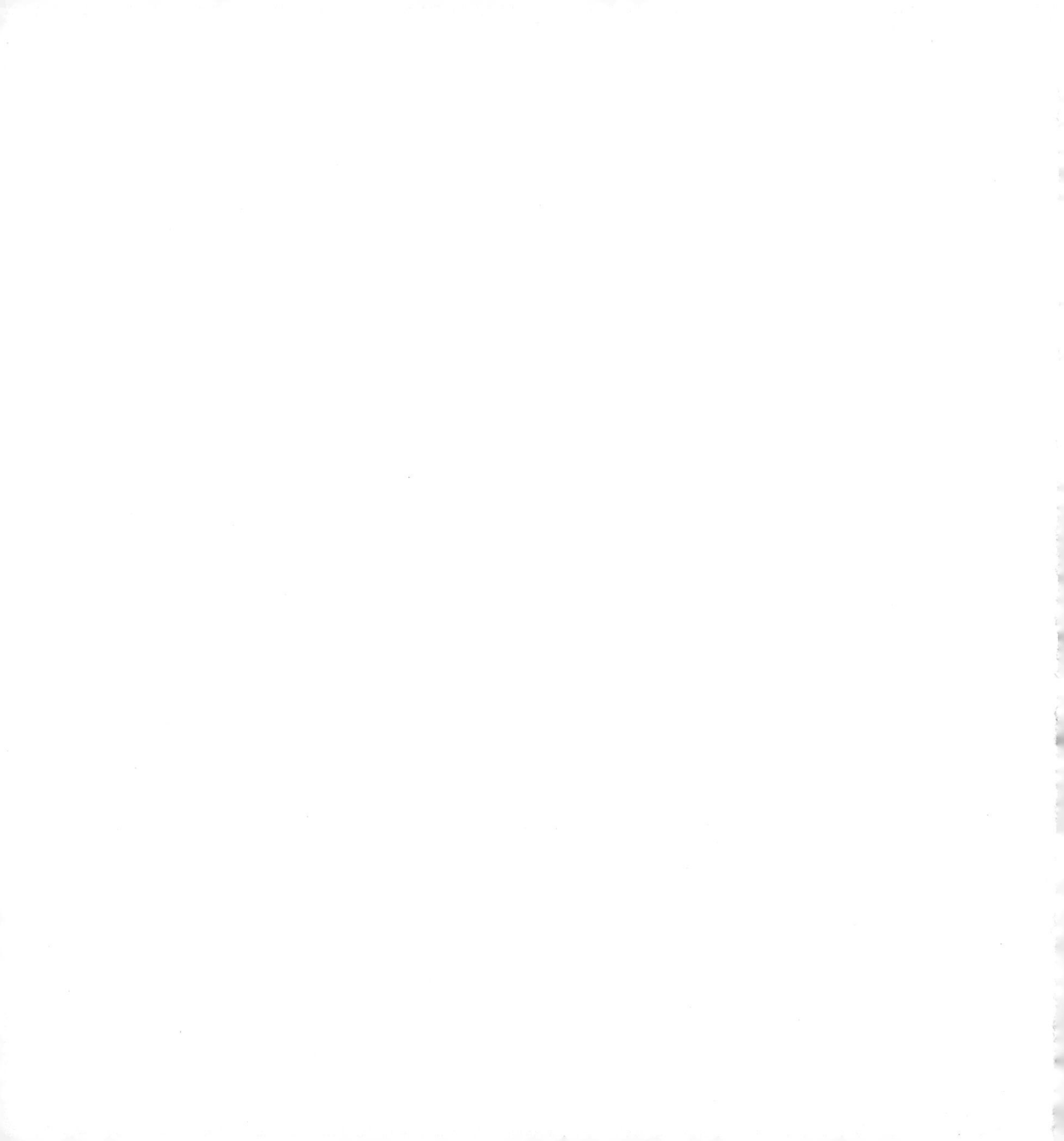